PRAISE FOR

I'LL DO IT MYSELF

Throughout life, we're sometimes lucky to meet people with a deep-seated passion for life. Sandra is most definitely one of these people; she lights up a room with just her presence. Her warm and loving nature would put a smile on the face of even the hardest of personalities. Sandra's story is sure to entertain and inspire.

COREY PITT
Area lead – Central Queensland, Australian Radio Network
arn.com.au

Just try to tell Sandra Hubert she can't do something – go on, I dare you. Sandra's story is nothing short of a remarkable journey revealing the strength of the human spirit. She has forged paths through obstacles that most people wouldn't contemplate, and in doing so reminds us that we are all stronger than we believe.

NATASHA BUTTLER, MBA-MCMR AMAMI CPM
Marketing strategist, Boost Marketing Services
boostmarketingservices.com.au

Sandra's story is engrossing and motivational in its message.

PETER WATT
Author
peterwatt.com

For anyone healing from a brain injury, there is no one roadmap for the journey to recovery. This is because each person – and each brain – is different. Sandra Hubert's beautiful memoir gives us not just a personal story; it also shows us the power of an individual to drive their own recovery. Through honesty, grit, resilience and humour, Sandra shows us what it looks like to take control of recovery and not simply accept the changes and challenges of a new life. This book is a terrific resource for anyone travelling along the same road who is looking for hope and inspiration.

LEE WOODRUFF
NYT best-selling author of In an Instant: A family's journey of love and healing
leewoodruff.com

I'll Do It Myself *is a compelling and inspiring read.*

Sandra and I have worked together many times over the years. She did an incredible job with the Australian Institute of Management in North Queensland. I have personally seen the contributions she has made to her family and in the community of North Queensland. Her commitment, passion and concern for others is infectious. Her efforts and achievements have been recognised by the business and broader community. I am indebted to her for her wisdom, good humour and support, in so many ways.

Her journey, determination and commitment following her illness have been truly amazing. She personifies her ethos of 'Live, laugh and love'.

I am honoured to endorse her book, and to acknowledge what a wonderful influence she has had on so many people. Her book will assist those who are facing challenges and adversity. She is a powerful role model and mentor to others.

GERARD BYRNE
MBA leadership program lecturer, James Cook University
gerardbyrne.com.au

Encephalitis (inflammation of the brain) is a thief. It has quietly been at work for hundreds of years, robbing families of their loved ones and often of the person they once knew. The injured brain can steal a person's capacity to remember, their personality and abilities many of us take for granted. For some, it can result in epilepsy and crippling fatigue. This is, of course, when the person survives – many don't.

When life gives you lemons, make lemonade ... Sandra Hubert is Chief Lemonade Maker! It is always heartening to hear a story of adversity overcome by such tenacity and determination. Sandra's story will be a comfort and inspiration to many facing hard times, whether it be from encephalitis or some other illness. Her most important words are perhaps those that open her first chapter: '... we forget to stop and smell the flowers.' A lesson for us all that living in the now is important; none of us knows what tomorrow holds.

DR AVA EASTON
Chief executive, Encephalitis International
encephalitis.info

Sandra's story is one of growth and rebuilding after the most tragic of experiences. As a reader you are brought into her world, and you will cry, smile and cheer as she beats the odds. She shares how she put the broken pieces of her life back together, just like a kintsugi bowl. You will see the gold glisten through the good that she brings to her community and the causes she feels so passionately about – and you will be left feeling inspired to rethink your own life.

RACHEL ALLAN
Entrepreneur, investor, coach & growth strategist
rachelallan.com.au

In print as in person, Sandra is inspirational. This work shines a wonderful spotlight on her never give in, never give up approach to life.

DAVID DONOHUE
Company director

In a world where people often mask who they really are, Sandra Hubert is a breath of fresh air. What you see (or read in this book) is what you get.

Sandra doesn't hold back from sharing the hard details of her brain injury and its even harder recovery. She does this because she genuinely wants to help people live better lives (I have seen this myself in her work for selectability Ltd).

I know you'll find yourself drawn into her story – Sandra's love, strength and enthusiasm almost leap off the pages!

DEBRA BURDEN, BBUS FIML FAICD
CEO, selectability Ltd
selectability.com.au

This beautiful book invites you on a journey. It takes you beyond the story of human suffering and peels back the layers to reveal the true strength and character that lies within us all, if we are willing to persist. Here is a power-filled line from Sandra's book: 'Life always seems better when you feel understood.'

JOANNE LYNAM
Author of An Angel at My Door: A mother's fight for her daughter to live to her potential
joannelynam.com

Sandra's story is one of courage, determination, resilience, growth, family and love. While reading it, I laughed, cried and punched the air! You, too, will be inspired as you follow her remarkable journey. I am honoured to be counted among Sandra's friends and when she says she is there for you ... she means it! I highly recommend this book – her suggestions and advice are relevant for everyone, regardless of injury, age or stage of life.

JENNIFER TELFER
Founder, Women of Worth (WOW) Townsville
facebook.com/groups/50035296712936

Owner, Dakini Bookbinding & Design
dakini.com.au

I first encountered Sandra's story when she submitted a chapter for my book Real Women, Real Stories. My heart is full of joy and gratitude to see her own beautiful book now in print.

When reading the deeper details of Sandra's story in this book, my eyes filled with tears and then with joy. What a journey she has been on. She is a woman of resilience, determination and absolute courage.

Sandra, you are a testament to what can happen when you decide to make the impossible possible. Thank you for sharing your story.

Reader, get ready – your life is about to be impacted beyond measure. You, too, will want to put your hands on your hips and say, 'I'll do it myself.' Allow Sandra's story to remind you that you have what it takes. There is nothing you can't achieve.

JENNIFER IRONSIDE
Master neurolinguistic emotional change practitioner and brain health trainer
jenniferironside.com

An uplifting story of the power of love and determination, Sandra's response to a debilitating brain injury will surely inspire readers to look at their own lives with a new perspective.

TONI LANPHIER
Archivist, The Cathedral School
cathedral.qld.edu.au

I'LL DO IT MYSELF

REBUILDING MY LIFE AFTER SERIOUS BRAIN INJURY

SANDRA HUBERT

First published in 2024 by Sandra Hubert
sandrahubert.com

© Sandra Hubert 2024

The moral rights of the author have been asserted.

All rights reserved. Except as permitted under international copyright laws, no part of this book may be reproduced in any form or by any means, be stored in a retrieval system, or be communicated or transmitted in any form or by any means, without prior written permission. All enquiries should be made to the publisher at the above website.

Publishing consultancy and editing: Publish in Style | publishinstyle.com
Cover design: Amy De Wolfe | amydewolfe.com
Author cover photos: Melanie Klaassen | wildfloraphotography.com.au
Interior design and layout: Amy De Wolfe | amydewolfe.com
Photo on page 209: News Ltd/Newspix

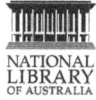 A catalogue record for this book is available from the National Library of Australia

ISBN: 9780645981605

Disclaimer

The author of this book does not dispense medical, psychological, financial, legal or business advice or prescribe the use of any technique as a form of treatment for associated problems without the advice of a relevant professional, either directly or indirectly. The intent of the author is only to offer information of a general nature to help you improve your life. In the event that you use the information in this book for yourself, the author assumes no responsibility for your actions. The views, thoughts and opinions expressed within this book belong solely to the author.

Contents

Dedication 11
Sandra's Snippets 13
A Note from Sandra 15

Chapter 1 17
Chapter 2 25
Chapter 3 35
Chapter 4 41
Chapter 5 49
Chapter 6 57
Chapter 7 69
Chapter 8 73
Chapter 9 83
Chapter 10 91
Chapter 11 97
Chapter 12 105
Chapter 13 109
Chapter 14 115
Chapter 15 121
Chapter 16 129
Chapter 17 133
Chapter 18 143
Chapter 19 147
Chapter 20 153
Chapter 21 159
Chapter 22 163
Chapter 23 169

Chapter 24	177
Chapter 25	179
Chapter 26	187
Chapter 27	197
Chapter 28	201
Chapter 29	207
Chapter 30	213
Chapter 31	223
Chapter 32	229
Chapter 33	231
Chapter 34	235
Chapter 35	237
Helpful Hints	239
Acknowledgements	249
About Sandra	255
Mentoring Magic	257

Dedication

I dedicate my book to my awesome husband Roland, who loves me totally and has always encouraged me to reach my goals. I also dedicate it to our three sons – Tyrnan, Kyle and Jaiden. Our sons have enriched our lives and shown us how wonderful it is to be a family.

You all never gave up on me, and you gave me reason to live. I thank you so much. Spending time together and seeing us all achieve our goals is a real blessing. I'll love you forever.

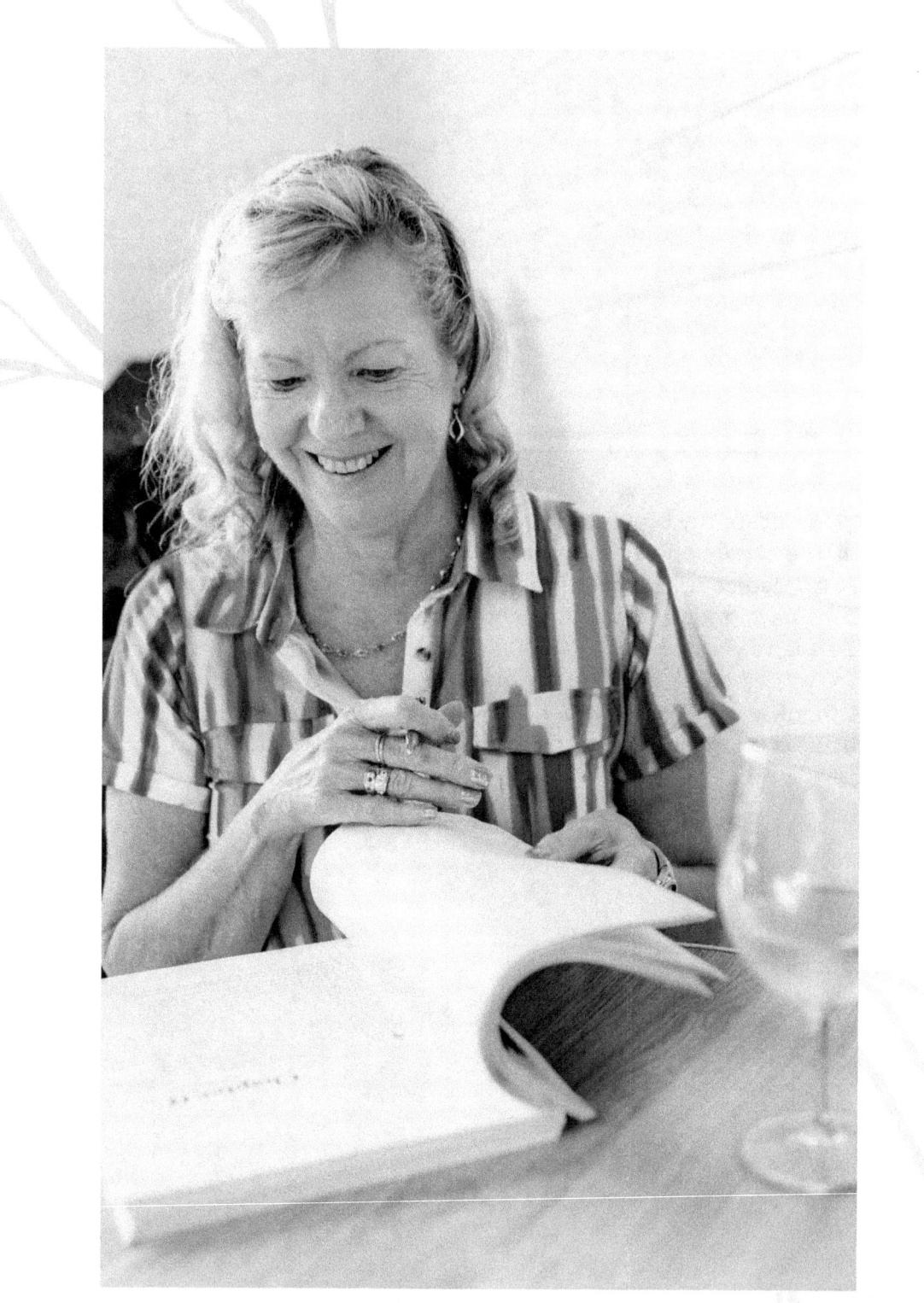

SANDRA'S SNIPPETS

Life always seems *better*
when you feel understood.

It also feels good when you have
a strong, positive person in your world.

When you read my story, you'll see how I nearly
died and had to rebuild my life – from that
experience, I created strategies for rebuilding.

I now share these
(and my love for people – and for life)
as often as I can.

If you'd like a loving dose of empathetic
wisdom and a good laugh,
head here to sign up for my regular
'Sandra's Snippets' emails:

sandrahubert.com

You only have one life.

Why not make it fun and happy,
despite the challenges?!

———

A Note from Sandra

Each of us treads a different path in life. As I look back on mine, I am humbled at what I have been through and how much I have achieved. I have always taken notes, asked questions, believed in myself and dreamed big. I didn't want to walk in someone else's footsteps. I wanted the strength to walk my own path but with a kind heart so that I could help others along the way.

I grew up in a world of fast cars and motorcycles and choices. My life has been filled with opportunities and good times, and with many adversities and rough times that physically and mentally challenged my strength. During these times I have often referred to the 'mantra for life' that my dad taught me as young girl:

1. Know your vehicle
2. Understand your limits
3. Be seen
4. Let people know what you are doing
5. Always make it home

I like lists and positive actions. So when my life fell apart after sustaining serious brain injury, I referred to my mantra for life and wrote a new list. I asked myself, 'What do I have? What can I do? What do I want to achieve? How can I achieve my goals?' I never gave up, even when the journey ahead seemed too hard. In the back of my mind I knew that I would, one day, write my story so that I could help and inspire others and hopefully make their journeys easier.

Recently I was chatting with my awesome psychologist, Christine. She asked me to look up the Japanese concept of kintsugi, because she could see parallels between that and what had happened with my brain. Kintsugi involves using gold lacquer to repair broken pieces of pottery. I love this analogy – we can embrace the broken pieces of our lives and choose to join them back together with gold, creating something beautiful and strong. If we think of the process in this way it allows us to celebrate our flaws and scars, stay optimistic when things fall apart, and embrace ourselves.

After my injury I made the decision to write that new list and rebuild my brain and my life, piece by piece. My hope is that you are inspired by my story to craft *your* life into a beautiful work of art, knowing that when challenges come, you can see the gold within them.

Sandra.

Chapter 1

Sometimes, we forget to stop and smell the flowers. However, when we become aware of what is happening around us, we often capture important memories for the future. As a child growing up in South Australia, I definitely lived in the moment. My fondest memories are those where I am with my older sister, spending wonderful moments with our grandparents. The laughter, the unconditional love, the learning together and the knowing that you can be anything you want to be ... those are my treasured memories. I was also a determined little person who often placed her hands on her hips and said, 'I'll do it myself.' This trait would go on to get me through many hard times.

Our family moved to Brisbane when I was six years of age, and it's there that the pace of our lives sped up. My dad was the Queensland state sales manager for Yamaha motorcycles, and he also became very involved in racing. Our weekends were spent at racetracks all over Queensland. We all had so much fun there and made many lifelong friendships. I remember being in the pits with the crew at each racetrack and taking drinks out to the flag men. We also used to help Mum at the checkpoints for Enduro racing (a type of fast-paced cross-country racing), which was always fun. The checkpoints were at the hill climbs, mud holes or creek crossings, so we saw lots of action.

At Easter, we always headed to the Bathurst track for motorcycle racing (this was back in the 1970s when they held races for

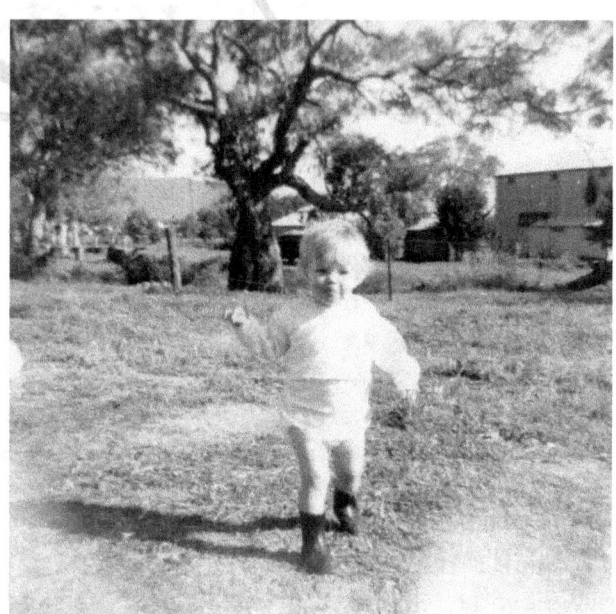
Little me, at about 20 months of age

CHAPTER 1

modified, supercharged bikes). My sister and I could tell the type of bike by its sound and we could guess the problem a bike was having when it came into the pits. This is where I learned that you have to know your vehicle and your limits and to make sure that you always make it home, just as my dad had taught me. When a rider has bike trouble and they make it back in order to have it fixed, there's a feeling of relief in the pits. It's the feeling that parents have when their children return home safely.

One of my dreams back then was to race motorbikes. My dad gave the late, great Gregg Hansford sponsorship with Yamaha at the start of Gregg's career. He was like a big brother to me and he once took me for a ride around the track. I was about 10 years of age and I was so excited. He told me to hold on, to do whatever he did and to not look down. Well, two out of three ain't bad ... Gregg knew that I had looked down when going around a corner because I flinched (something that is natural to do because the road is so close to your knee). This ride cured me from ever going into racing – give me a car, any day!

So, at a young age, I could ride a bike, but I could also drive dune buggies and four-wheelers. My sister and I were pretty self-sufficient and learned how to fix things ourselves while our parents were out riding. Dad also gave us skills in defensive driving and car maintenance. When teaching us to drive, Dad would tell us to be aware of our surroundings and he would role play incidents. For example, he would say, 'You've blown a tyre. Show me what you'd do.' He wanted to make us respond quickly and be safe in any situation. He said that he only had one chance to protect us, and that was by teaching us well. Because we pretty much grew up on a racetrack, we were used to a fast pace and were aware of many dangers. It made me realise that life is like a racetrack – when you're at the starting line of any journey, be aware of your surroundings, breathe and relax, and then get ready, get set ... and go.

We also had great family friends, the Powells, who lived across the road. We holidayed together and were there for each other in happy and sad times. Growing up, mum would tell us that if we had any problems, we should ring Mr and Mrs Powell, and I knew their phone number off by heart. I really did have a fabulous childhood in Brisbane, one that let me experience life and appreciate the value of life.

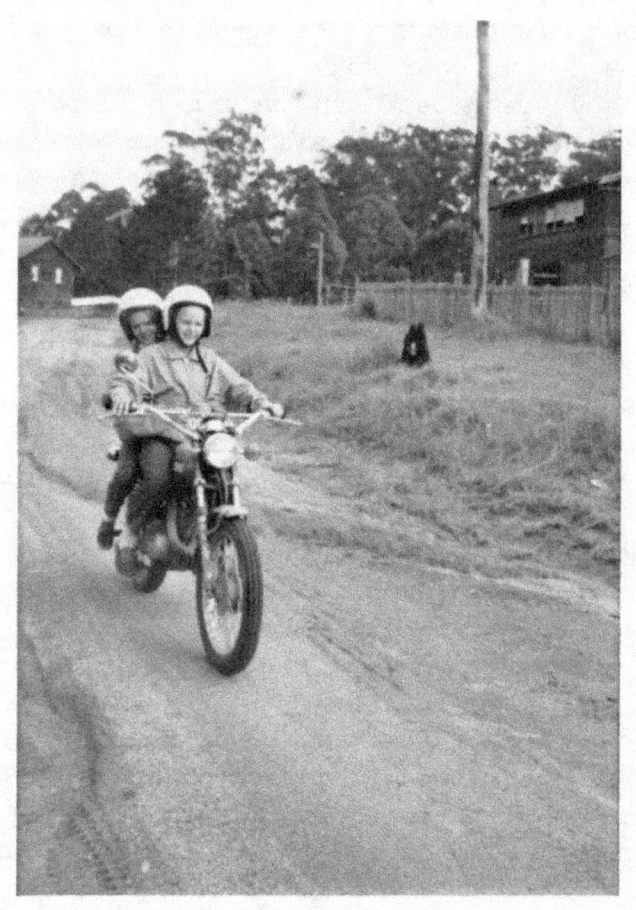

Joanne and me in 1972, aged 12 and 9

CHAPTER 1

When I was 11 years of age, our family once again moved. This time it was to sunny Townsville in north Queensland. My dad bought a Yamaha motorcycle dealership and started his own racing team. Our lives revolved around motorcycle racing again, and I was ready to start high school. It wasn't until then that we realised I needed glasses for long-distance vision. I didn't understand why I couldn't see properly – no one in our family was short-sighted. I have great coping skills, and all of my life I had learned how to make people believe I was just like them (that is, a person with normal vision). I used other methods to find things out. For example, when I couldn't see the items listed on a menu on a wall, I would ask a friend what they were having from the menu. I also coped by being very friendly to people because from a distance I couldn't identify who they were – only when they were close enough could I see them clearly.

It was my awesome Poppa who picked up on my short-sightedness. When he and my grandma visited for the Christmas holidays just after we moved to Townsville, they took us out for ice cream. He asked me what ice cream I'd like, and he watched me. Remember me mentioning that my grandparents gave me unconditional love and protected me? Well, my Poppa saw me squint and then ask my sister what she was having. Poppa turned to me and asked what I could see on the board that was hanging from the ceiling. I told him politely what I could see – the Peters and Streets symbols. He turned to my mum, placed a protective arm around me, and in a stern voice that I had never heard before, pointed at my mum and said, 'My granddaughter can't see properly. You take her to the doctor and get her glasses.' It was like a light came on. Mum stood there, blinking. I think she was in disbelief. She said, 'I will.' I stood there feeling taller because I realised that I had a vision problem and that it was going to be fixed. Plus, my Poppa would make sure that it happened.

When I put on those new glasses ... wow. The world looked amazing. I could see tree leaves and flowers. I could see planes and helicopters (not just hear them). I could read the signs on the side of the road (not just guess at what they said). I loved my new glasses and appreciated all the little things I saw. If anybody at school tried to make fun of me for wearing glasses, I'd say, 'I can see better and more than you can.' It made them start wondering what they were missing out on. It's all about how you present yourself – the way you

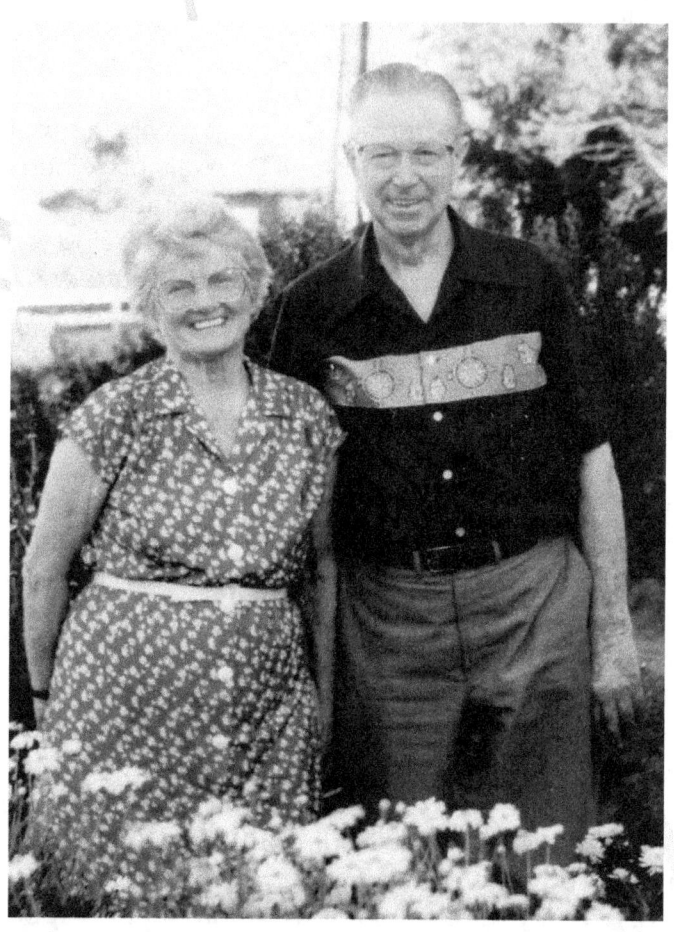
My beloved Grandma and Poppa in 1987, in their front yard in South Australia

CHAPTER 1

hold up your head and look the world in the eye. Let people wonder why you are smiling!

I made some incredible friendships as a teenager, with many of them becoming just like family. They are still so important in my life. I send a big 'thank you' to them all. We have been there for each other so many times, and I feel that it is important to have a support group – be it friends or family. I was lucky to have a special group of friends that I saw every week. We went roller-skating and to the movies, and drove four hours (each way) in one day to Cairns to go on waterslides. All of our mums made us food when we visited each other's homes to play pool, swim, play board games or watch movies together. We'd go to cafes, sit together and chat, or drive down the Strand (Townsville's esplanade) to catch up with other friends. We knew each other's families and even fixed each other's cars. We had fun riding motorcycles and going four-wheel-driving, fishing and camping. We celebrated birthdays together and looked out for each other. I have *so* many happy memories.

One special friend, Craig, really is family to me. Over the years we would sit and chat for hours and help each other with any problems. His mum and dad opened their home to me, and often we would all sit in the loungeroom enjoying a cuppa. When Craig broke his foot while at technical college in Brisbane, it only took a phone call for four of us to jump into a car and drive the 1360 kilometres to pick up his car and then turn around and drive home (Craig was flown home). When Craig and I get together the conversation usually starts with 'Remember when?' His friendship will last forever and it (along with the memories) would help me so much in later years.

(Note: If you haven't been to Townsville, you really should visit. It's such a great place because within a couple of hours' drive you can be at the Great Barrier Reef, the outback or a rainforest.)

I met a lovely young man called Scott just before my 17th birthday. He became my first boyfriend and we are still good friends. He introduced me to the music of Phil Collins, who is still my favourite singer – I *love* his music. Music is so important to many of us; when you hear a song, the memory of where you heard it comes back to you. Back then, my friends and I loved roller-skating to music that had a good beat – it got us all in a happy mood. Also, each of my friends played different music in their cars. For example, when we got into Barry's car, we'd say, 'Shall we listen to Anne Murray, Anne Murray or

Anne Murray?' We would then smile and laugh together as we drove off listening to Anne Murray (I'm smiling at this memory right now!). Hearing Phil Collins' music makes me remember places and times when I was healthy and happy. 'In the Air Tonight' is my favourite. Whenever I hear it, I am instantly a teenager again in a car with my friends, with all of us laughing. When the drum solo finished, we knew exactly how long to hold the rewind button on the cassette player so that we could hear it again and again. How could I have known back then that these memories would be so important in years to come?

———————

Chapter 2

Do you believe in fate? I do. One evening when I was 17 years of age, we had two parties to go to; one was at my best friend Susan's house and the other was at my boyfriend's sister's house. We chose to go to Susan's party first. A young man called Roland was at Susan's party and when he saw me walk in he said to himself, 'One day, I'm going to marry that girl.' However, before Roland (who did, indeed, marry me four years later) could be introduced to me, my boyfriend and I left to go to the second party. In the years after that there were so many times when our paths nearly crossed. Once, my friends and I had been four-wheel-driving up Hervey Range (as we often did), and it rained heavily. Coming home we had to cross Keelbottom Creek, and water was starting to flow across the road. It usually had non-flowing water across it, and we knew the crossing very well. So, the guys just put tarps over the fronts of the two cars and we went in convoy, slowly, across the creek. There was a car on the other side of the creek so we figured that if something happened, the occupants could help us. Little did we know that my future husband was in that car.

It was three years later when I discovered that Roland had been in that car. He and I were driving up Hervey Range. It was raining and I was reminded of the creek crossing. I mentioned it to Roland, and a quizzical look came across his face. He raised his eyebrows and said, 'That was you!' I said, 'Yes.' We shook our heads, not believing how close we had come to meeting way back then.

Roland and I ended up meeting through a mutual friend. If you're about my age and you know Townsville, then you know that in the '80s the Strand was the meeting place for all of us teenagers. We parked down there, walked along the beach and chatted for hours. After going out at night, we'd all go for a 'lappy'. This was a drive along the Strand to see who was out and about and to catch up. In 1983, at the age of 20, I was chatting with my good mate Wayne on the Strand when Roland, the guy from three years previous who had said to himself that 'he'd marry me', drove past and saw us. Wayne was also Roland's friend, so Roland finally got the opportunity to meet me. It was up to him to make a good impression. I immediately noticed his beautiful blue eyes, and his lovely smile (which made me smile even more). There was an instant connection. When he left, I hoped that I would see him again. Wayne still asks me if I have forgiven him for introducing Roland to me. Gotta love good friends.

To this day, my husband and I still go for a lappy along the Strand. We may not see anyone we know from the old days while on the drive, but we reminisce about our youth ... and we believe that if we stop going for a lappy, we're getting old. (Do you have any rituals that you like to do so that you keep feeling young?)

Remember me saying earlier that I had really good friends whom I could trust? Well, it seems that maybe I was mistaken about them being trustworthy! Why? Because behind my back, they wanted to play matchmaker. After Roland and I met, he seemed to turn up wherever I was, without me telling him of my plans. It seems that another mutual mate, Peter, liked playing Cupid. Once – when we were all at a café having a cuppa and milkshake after roller-skating – Peter made sure that Roland didn't have a car so that he would need a lift home. My friends know how caring I am and that I would help out, and Roland's house was on my way home. So, when we were getting ready to leave, Peter (acting all innocent) asked who could drop Roland home. Like a script in a play, I put up my hand and offered to do it. It was years before I found out that Peter had played Cupid.

Revenge is sweet, especially when you take your time to repay it. I found my opportunity 16 years later at Peter's wedding reception. Roland was MC at the wedding, so it was easy to have a 'summons' be served when the telegrams were being read. I was the 'spitefully aggrieved' under the Mates Act of Queensland,

I must admit that I didn't make it easy for Roland to ask me out.

Regulation U R Nought Y, Section C. In the summons, the judge had ruled that Peter had to continue his Cupid-like actions for the rest of his life. I had a police friend help me to write it, and Peter and his beautiful wife Louise had it framed. They loved it.

I must admit that I didn't make it easy for Roland to ask me out. However, persistence pays off, as they say. A few weeks after I dropped off Roland at his house, he turned up at my workplace and asked for my phone number. I was so nervous that I just told him that my number was in the phonebook. When I hopped into my car to drive home, I realised that my parents had moved and the phonebook featured their old address. Oops. However, Roland remembered that Wayne and I had mentioned that we were neighbours, so he decided to drive around Wayne's suburb to find my car. Unfortunately, he didn't realise that although we both lived out of town on the north side, we were not in the same suburb. Roland was persistent – he tried driving around the next suburb, and found my car. He looked up the address and this led to finding my phone number ... which meant he could then ring me and ask me out! By going to such lengths to find my phone number, at least I knew he was serious. When he rang and asked me out, I was on cloud nine. How could I not say, 'Yes'?

Dads can be protective, can't they? Well, my dad was. I recall the first time Roland drove up our driveway. Dad said in a stern voice, 'Who's that driving down my driveway?' I did a little skip and said in an excited tone, 'It's for me!' Mum saw my reaction and said, 'This one is trouble.' She meant this in a nice way because she hadn't seen that type of reaction from me before. Mum knew straight away that this boy was special.

On our first couple of dates, I did everything I could *not* to let Roland hold my hand. He tried so many times. Somehow, I knew that once I gave him my hand, it would be for life. After a lovely evening out, while Roland was driving me home, I placed my hand near his. Roland placed his hand on mine – and he still holds my hand today.

Here's an extract from my diary, written a couple of months after our first date:

This diary is just my collection of events that happened after meeting Roland. I have not known him a long time. He fills my heart with love, my life with joy. So I am writing this so that all

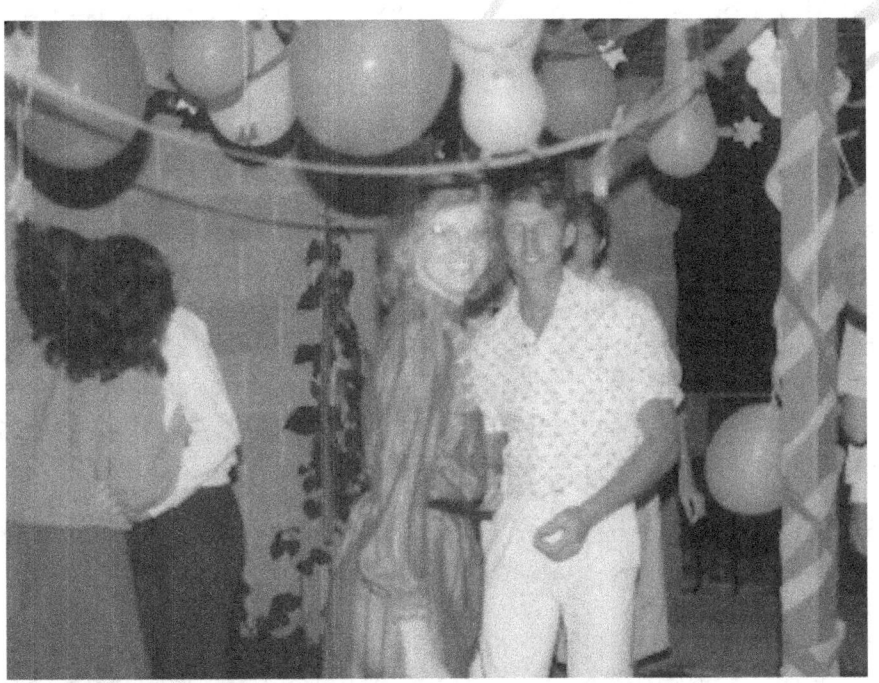
Dancing the night away with Roland at my 21st birthday party

my memories can be kept and reread all the days of my life. I can share my thoughts, my feelings and my life. To Roland. To my love, my life, to be with you forever. Love Sandra xo

I love writing diary entries, and I think this love must come from my nan (my dad's mum). Nan wrote a diary for her entire married life. It is fascinating to read. Here's one entry, from 4 March 1958: *'Queen mother arrived in Adelaide. Waikerie organised a floral display and the helpers were Nan, Stella Boxall, Doris Thompson, Eileen Hawkes, Syd Rainey.'* My birth is announced in her diary, as are those of her other grandchildren. I have sometimes used wall calendars, business diaries and personal journals to record the events and feelings of my life, and little did I know that these records would one day help me to put the pieces of my life back together.

Roland and I discovered we had something in common – we both loved motor racing. I'd come from motorcycle racing and Roland from off-road racing and we both loved four-wheel-driving. A few months into our relationship, a mud car race was scheduled to be held at Townsville's Keyatta Park, so we decided to enter (with me as navigator). The course saw us drive down into the mud, go around five corners and then turn back, driving between two barrels at the finish line. We were the overall winners of three races, and spectators yelled out that it looked easy to do the course blindfolded. The marshals asked for nominations to race blindfolded. Roland and I looked at each other and said, 'It's now or never,' and up went our hands to confirm that we'd take up the challenge. Hey, we were young and invincible (this was before we had children!). Roland was blindfolded by one of the marshals and I said to him, 'You know the track. I will tell you where the witches' hats are, which way to turn and which way you are sliding.' My only worry was making sure Roland had the car lined up straight so that we could get up the bank and through the barrels at the finish line. I yelled the information and directions and Roland did exactly as I told him. Oh wow – we did it, and we won! We trusted each other, and who wouldn't want to marry a man who did everything you told him to do? (I should add that this was the only time when he has done exactly what I have asked him to do.)

Roland and I were inseparable, always holding hands or touching our feet under the table. Six months after our first date, on the 15th anniversary of the moon landing, Roland proposed to me

CHAPTER 2

– on bended knee – at a restaurant while we were having dinner. We were oblivious of anyone else in the room but the staff and other patrons must have seen it all happen because they were quick to congratulate us. I was floating on air. When I got home, I jumped on my dad to wake him up to tell him the good news and flash my engagement ring.

Next up: wedding plans and looking for a place to call home. There were so many wonderful things to look forward to. I had dreamt of getting married and having children and I was seeing that dream come true. However, during this time my parents split up. I had to cope with this and become a go-between. Once again, I became that little girl with hands on hips, saying, 'I'll do it myself.' I told them both that they were my parents so they had to grow up and act like parents for my big day. They did do this, and I thank them for it. Dad walked me down the aisle on 2 December 1984, and Mum stood up at the end of the aisle to join us – this meant they could both give me away. At the reception my parents even danced together, arm in arm, for me. For that moment, my family was complete again.

My parent's separation gave me a real-life lesson in the importance of communicating and remaining true to yourself. This is so important. Roland and I have always taken time for each other and supported each other's goals and life journeys. We are very close – we touch when we go to sleep, even if it's only our feet touching. We have learned one good lesson and that is, 'Do not go to sleep holding hands, with your fingers entwined.' Why? Well, it cuts the circulation to your fingers and hurts so much when trying to separate them! Stop smiling. Have you done this, too? We laugh at this memory.

We had a couple of friends say that our marriage wouldn't last a year because we were total opposites. Roland was a bricklayer who had left school after grade 10. I had graduated year 12 and received an academic award for accounting and a school prize for community service, and I had also graduated university as an accountant. Why does it matter that we were different in that way? We were both hard-working people who enjoyed the same things and we thought the same way about life. To this day, we are two individuals who love living together and we both want the other to achieve their goals. There will always be people who try to knock you down, but this only makes me more determined.

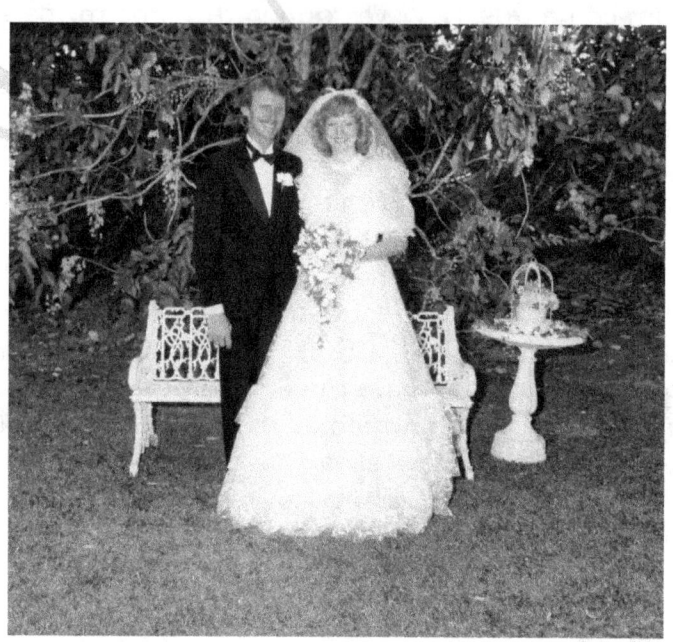
Our beautiful wedding day, 2 December 1984

CHAPTER 2

I'm a bit of a romantic, so I make sure we celebrate every anniversary, whether it be for our first date, our engagement, our wedding, Valentine's Day or birthdays. I also make sure that on every seventh wedding anniversary (so, the seventh, 14th, 21st, 28th etc anniversaries) we do something special or have a night away. We do this to cure that seven-year itch. Well, you can't be too careful, and it's a fun reminder to keep our love alive. We've told people that we are newlyweds and they say, 'Oh, isn't that lovely?' Roland's parents were married 68 years and we're nowhere near that yet.

Now, you might wonder how we keep the romance going. Well, our philosophy is that life is a journey, and that you can choose to make your journey memorable and enjoyable. It's important to make your loved one feel special. When Roland is out longer than normal or not home at the usual time, instead of getting cranky I send him a funny text or leave a voice message. It could be something like, 'Is this the classifieds? I'd like to put up an ad: "Hot woman looking for hot man for fun times. Only a married man need apply."' It's not what you say; it's the message that counts. A quick reply from him might be 'At Jack's, will be home in 20 min.' I know Roland would be smiling at my message and also thinking, 'Oh, shit, I forgot to let her know I was popping over to Jack's before coming home.' It's the way you do things that makes the difference. In that example, I found out where my husband was and when he'd be home, all without getting angry or upset. Oh, and there is always a hug when he arrives home. We read somewhere that hugs need to be at least 10 seconds long. So, we tried doing that and it does make a difference. Go on, give it a go – time yourself!

I worked as an accountant up until the birth of our first child, and then I worked with my husband for the first four years of motherhood, doing all his bookwork. These were great years. I loved working together, and I'd take the boys to have lunch with their dad on the job site. They knew to ask Daddy if they could play in the sand, just in case it had been treated with chemicals. They also knew to step carefully over the string lines and to help Daddy by getting his water bottle or bringing him a tool that he needed. Roland worked hard and we did what we could to have special times together as a couple. I used to get up early to cook Roland a big breakfast and make his lunch.

Being a romantic, I often put love notes in Roland's lunch box. That did make for some interesting conversations at work in front of the other guys! When Roland told me about his day and that he had found a note in his lunch box, I would smile and raise my eyebrows cheekily, saying, 'Wives do that!' He would give me a big smile and a cuddle. What I really loved about Roland was that he made me feel special and he wasn't shy about it. He would hold my hand in public, sometimes open the car door for me and even kiss me goodbye on a jobsite in front of everyone. He was my protector (like my Poppa had been) and my best friend. We'd do things like fix the car together and laugh when I'd pick the problem or solution before he did.

Chapter 3

I went back to full-time employment after the birth of our second child, as I needed to get my career as an accountant back on track. I also returned to study because I wanted to obtain my CPA (Certified Practising Accountant) and tax agent qualifications. Roland supported my career decision and enjoyed seeing me achieve. When Mummy was doing her assignments, our two sons thought she was drawing with them as we all sat at the table. These were special moments of time spent together. I worked for a couple of tax agents and enjoyed this work, especially in 1988 when the Australian Tax Office had a tax amnesty (meaning you could lodge previous years' returns without penalties). The highest number of returns I did for one person covered 20 years of returns. I had to do research for each year's return – it was fascinating to delve into so much tax history.

I'm very left-brain strong and I love numbers. I also love statistics and enjoy using numbers and percentages in my working and home lives. I am one of those people who remembers number plates, phone numbers, birthdates and special dates. I love playing card games because I count the cards and remember their order, which helps me predict the likelihood of each next card. When out on the road, I count cars and analyse the way they drive to ensure I choose the best lane. Numbers are my life.

After the tax-agent work I decided to go into management accounting. I found my dream job working for a large multi-national business with branches all over Australia. I looked after three of these branches. This was in the days before the internet, meaning that I had to wait for the mailman to deliver a floppy disc from each branch before I could enter their data into my computer. This computer was connected to our head office via a one-purpose line. I had deadlines to meet, and I remember pleading with one particular floppy disc and computer to work so that I could prepare the monthly accounts. I think I even said that I would marry the computer if it worked. The things we say when we are desperate ... What have you ever said to your computer or phone? Technology, huh?!

Have you ever found a job that is totally you? This position of management accountant stretched my mind and helped me achieve my personal goals. I worked with our state and head offices, travelling to each of my branch offices every second month. I had a great working relationship with my branch managers and general managers. I even had a visit from our general manager from England after I queried the way a new computer system was going to be implemented. It was a good meeting, with me outlining my concerns and offering ideas for a less-disruptive roll-out of the system. He liked my ideas and they were implemented. The staff were also happy with the outcome.

Here I was in my dream job, married to an awesome man, with a lovely home, great friends and two fantastic sons, and I was about to turn 30. It was a good time to reflect on my life. I felt a strong motherly feeling kick in, with a desire for our family to grow to three or four children. I loved those old western movies where brothers look out for each other – a third child would give our boys another playmate. Roland and I discussed it and decided that we would never regret having another baby. So, by the time my 31st birthday came around, we were happily expecting our third child.

I wanted to make the pregnancy announcement at Christmas lunch, but we all know that good plans sometimes change. We were in Brisbane at my dad's place. Breakfast was ready and my dad offered my sister and I a glass of Champagne. Of course, I declined, and to my surprise Dad became concerned because he'd never known me to say no to a Champagne breakfast. So, I had to tell him and my sister straight away that I was pregnant. He was so happy for us. Then I rang Mum, and after giving her lots of hints, such as by asking, 'How good is your knitting?', I had to just tell her. 'Mum I'm pregnant!' Her reply floored us: 'OK, I'll have to go now and digest

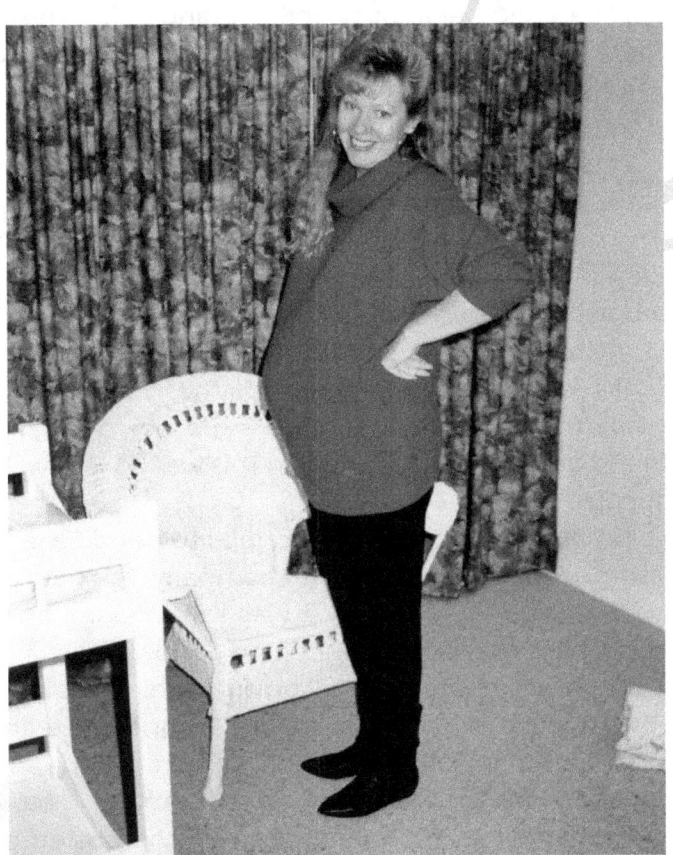

About seven months' pregnant with Jaiden, just before our nightmare began

this. I'll ring you back.' She then hung up. Dad and my sister looked at me. I was totally stunned and we all started laughing. There was going to be a seven-year gap between our second child and our third child, so I can see why Mum wasn't expecting that news. She called back after about 30 minutes, and was very excited about the prospect of another grandchild. I remember how excited she had been when I had told her about her first grandchild – she'd jumped around, squealing with joy and excitement. So, you can imagine how confused I was by her initial response to the news of my third child!

I went to the same obstetrician I had gone to with my previous baby, and Dr S was very happy with my pregnancy and progress. I applied for 52 weeks of maternity leave and was going to work right up until my due date because I had delivered late with my other pregnancies. My bosses were very happy for me and we discussed my work choices for when I returned from maternity leave. They also organised my replacement. Everything was going along smoothly. As the weeks went by, we prepared for the little addition to our family. We didn't know if we were having a boy or a girl, and my dear girlfriend gave me a baby shower. This was a first for me, which made it special.

By this time, Roland had changed jobs to get off the tools and was a salesman for a building supplies company. This gave him more time to be with our children and it was less stressful on his body. Now he could stay awake when watching a movie!

My work commitments were full on as I readied my branches for my impending leave. When I was heavily pregnant, we attended a few functions for Roland's work. Our neighbours – Bruce and Sharon – were the best and were always willing to jump the fence any time we needed a babysitter. My weekly visits to the obstetrician were going well. With three weeks to go, I started to get headaches at the back of my head. They were really bad but I put them down to working hard to get end-of-month tasks done before I went on maternity leave. I was going to the toilet often but in the latter stage of pregnancy you tend to do that. I had been fine at my previous doctor's visit and I only had a few days before my next visit so I just did my best to cope with the really bad headaches.

At the end of my workday on Wednesday 3 August 1994, with only two weeks until my due date, I drove home tired and with a headache. I went along Nathan Street, which is a long, straight road.

> *With three weeks to go,
> I started to get headaches
> at the back of my head.*

I'LL DO IT MYSELF

When I needed to turn right, I could see a green turning arrow, but because my headache was so bad I didn't check the lights again as I came closer and made the turn. As I turned, I realised that I had run a red light and three lanes of traffic were coming towards me. I got through the intersection unscathed, and it wasn't a close call, but it shook me up a bit because I'm such a careful driver. Roland had a work function that night but I declined to go because my headache had become so bad – also, I felt warmer than usual. I put all of this down to being tired and heavily pregnant. Little did I know that this would be my last day at work, and also the last day of me (as I knew me). It was going to be the start of a journey for which I would need every ounce of strength and determination. The ride of a lifetime.

———

Chapter 4

At about 5am on Thursday 4 August 1994, Roland woke to find me having a fit in bed. He panicked and immediately called 000. Instead of waiting for the operator to connect him to the ambulance operator, he yelled out, 'I need an ambulance now! My wife is having a fit and she is very pregnant.' He rattled off our address and hung up to attend to me. Minutes passed but it seemed like hours, and no ambulance had arrived so Roland rang 000 again. As he started to repeat everything, the operator calmly asked, 'What house number are you?' Roland was flustered and quickly replied, '19.' He heard her say the number and then heard the ambulance pull up in our driveway. The operator explained that she didn't catch the number the first time or have time to transfer him to an ambulance operator. She said that the ambulance had been in our street looking for us, and a second one was on its way.

The paramedics came straight inside to attend to me, and the second ambulance arrived with its sirens blaring. This noise attracted the attention of our awesome neighbours Bruce and Sharon, who ran straight outside expecting only happy baby news. Instead, they were faced with the seriousness of the situation. The paramedics said that although the fit was over, I was still 'out of it'. To calm Roland, they told him that the cause was more than likely high blood pressure. I was placed on the trolley and readied for transport to the hospital. Bruce told Roland to get in the ambulance with me because he and Sharon would look after everything. Sharon ran inside to be with our two sons, then aged seven and nine. She had often babysat the boys and looked after our home and animals when we'd gone away on holidays over the previous six years.

The second ambulance had been called because they wanted another paramedic to be in the back of the ambulance with me, in case I had another fit. Roland was worried because I had high blood pressure, but the ambulance officer tried to calm him by telling him that this was normal and that I should be OK. Off we went to Park Haven Private Hospital, arriving at 7am.

By the time we got to the hospital, I was aware of my surroundings, but feeling drowsy. Because I was 38 weeks' pregnant, they took me to the maternity ward. My obstetrician, Dr S, met us there and did an examination. At every appointment throughout the pregnancy, I had been healthy and without problems. He knew straight away that there was an issue because although my blood pressure was fine, I had a temperature, pale skin, neck discomfort and back pain, and I was fidgety. He started an IV line straight away and called a neurologist – Dr R – to come immediately.

Dr R did his review and asked for a CT scan and more blood tests. I spoke to both Dr R and Dr S and answered their questions as though nothing was wrong with me, but they knew better. Roland asked them, 'Why did Sandra have a fit?' Dr R's calm reply was, 'You can have one fit for no reason at all.' Roland then asked if I would be likely to have another one. Dr R said that he didn't know, but he would have someone with me all the time to look after me.

By 10.30am I had been to the X-ray department for a CT scan, and had had blood tests. They also put me on an IV of anti-seizure medication. Throughout the afternoon my temperature was still high, yet they couldn't bring it down. At 3.15pm I was also still complaining of headaches and they noticed that I was starting to get a bit wobbly on my feet when I walked to the toilet.

Roland had been by my side all day, talking with me and telling me how much he loved me. When I was comfortably settled in my room, the nurse told Roland that she had to go to the toilet. She asked him if he wanted another nurse to be called in or if he would be OK alone with me for a few minutes. He is my protector so, of course, he said, 'It's fine, I'll be OK.'

The nurse left and we were finally alone. I looked up at him and said, 'I'm scared.' Roland held my hand and said that he was scared,

CHAPTER 4

too – and it was then that I had another seizure. Roland pressed the button and yelled down the corridor, 'I need help!' Nurses came from everywhere to attend to me. Roland was beside himself with worry. My seizure was timed and it was decided that I had experienced a grand mal-type seizure. Dr S and Dr R were informed of this, and Dr R came straight in and checked me again. He wasn't sure what was causing my high temperature, which had led to the seizure. He wanted to put me on a broad spectrum of antibiotics straight away and for me to have another CT scan and a lumbar puncture. The nurses cleaned me up, brushed my hair and settled me in before sending me for the scans and tests.

When I was ready to go for my scans, the nurses asked Roland – who had been at my side all day and was showing signs of exhaustion – if he'd like to go home for a while and have a rest. They would phone him if there was any change in my condition. Roland said that he would go home but return with our sons. No one could give Roland any answers and he was so worried that his beautiful wife would die. He wanted our sons to spend some time with their mummy ... in case it was the last time they got to do so.

Roland arrived home and it was the first time he had had a moment to think or to call anyone. He rang my dad in Brisbane, who was expecting the usual 'Happy Birthday' phone call from his daughter. Instead, he heard, 'Your daughter is in hospital ... I'll ring you back.' He then rang my mum, in South Australia, to tell her all that he knew. He suspected she may have already felt that something was wrong. Mum said she would organise a flight to come up. The other call Roland made was to our dear friends Pete and Sonia, who were also expecting a baby. Pete (a different Peter to the one I mentioned in chapter 2) and I had been friends since we were about 14 years of age and I often called him my twin brother because we were born 10 days apart (however, he is older than me – and I remind him of this all the time!). Roland and Pete had become really good friends, and right then Roland needed a friend. At the end of their call, Pete said Roland could call at any time, and they sent their love and support to me.

By 6pm Dr R had performed my lumbar puncture and had instructed nurses that I was to lie flat for 12 hours. The results of the lumbar puncture were to be phoned to Dr R as soon as possible because he suspected that I had either viral or bacterial meningitis.

Both Dr S and Dr R kept checking on me and ordered an IV featuring high doses of antibiotics. My doctors were doing their best to stabilise me and to work out what I had. My life was in their hands.

Roland arrived back at the hospital with our two boys, who wanted to see their loved mummy. I was set up in my room on a drip and looked OK. It took a little while for the boys to understand what was going on, but at least we had cuddles and time together. I spoke with everyone and my condition seemed to be under control. Roland was still very concerned but he had to take the boys home, so he kissed me goodbye and told me he'd be back in the morning.

In the early hours of Friday morning, the nurses let the doctors know that my temperature still hadn't come down and my headaches were worse (especially at the back of my head when I moved it). At about 7am Dr R made the decision to move me out of maternity into isolation and to treat my condition as bacterial meningitis. He also prescribed 10 days of IV antibiotics. By 9am I was settled in my new room. Dr R gave strict instructions that I was a special patient and needed 24/7 care. Roland had rung the hospital and was told that I was sleeping most of the time, that I still had a headache and that I appeared to know where I was and what was happening.

Our neighbours fed the boys and took them to school. Roland went to his boss to explain the situation and to ask for his holidays to be brought forward. His boss was very supportive and sent best wishes for my recovery. Roland also called in to see his elderly parents and let them know what was happening. They came up to see me. Roland's mum was very health aware and we lovingly called her a witch doctor. She had a remedy for everything and it always worked. When she walked in, she knew something wasn't right with me. The way I looked scared her and although she gave us her love and support, she quickly left the room, upset.

My condition was deteriorating rapidly and by 3.30pm I was moved to my own room for safety reasons, in case I was contagious (at that stage they still didn't know what I had). Everyone would have to wear masks and coats in this room, and gloves for personal contact. My temperature still hadn't come down and they had tried almost everything. They had to be careful because I was heavily pregnant – they feared for our unborn child. Roland stayed with me till the evening because he was so worried. He held my hand and talked with me. At about 5.30pm I became more fidgety so

CHAPTER 4

Dr R changed my antibiotics. Dr S also attended. At about 9pm Dr R was notified that I was getting more confused and fidgety so he ordered a sedative to calm me. By 10pm I wasn't sure who Roland was, which was so distressing for him. Dr R came back in and the CT scan results arrived.

They showed that it was likely that I had viral meningitis or viral encephalitis. Dr R said to continue IV antibiotics plus start an IV of acyclovir because he suspected that, due to the severity of my case, it was more than likely that I had viral encephalitis. Another CT scan was ordered for the morning. Dr R was still in my room at 11pm when I had a seizure. Roland and the nurse settled me down and I was given a sedative to help but then I had another seizure, followed by another one. It was decided that I needed intensive care. Townsville General Hospital (as it was then known) was called but we were told that its ICU was full.

The medical staff thought they had my seizures under control, but I had another grand mal seizure at 1am (on 6 August), and the nurses asked Roland to leave the room. This panicked Roland, who had had no sleep and was in emotional turmoil because the love of his life was suffering in front of him. A nurse asked if there was someone he could call for support. Roland rang Pete, who jumped out of bed, got dressed and raced up to the hospital. By 2am Dr R had assessed me and called for an anaesthetist because they needed to stop the seizures; they were now almost continuous and I wasn't recovering between them. The anaesthetist sedated me enough to stop the seizures but not harm the baby. Dr R then had discussions with Dr S and it was decided that I needed to be in intensive care *now*. I would have to be transferred immediately to Townsville General Hospital – they would just have to make room for me there.

It was decided that I should give birth to my baby, and then be placed in an induced coma to stop the seizures and give my brain time to heal. Dr S is a private doctor, who usually does not perform surgery in a public hospital, but he said that he would deliver our baby by emergency caesarean at the general hospital. Dr R could then place me in a coma, which would give doctors more control and a better chance of helping me to recover. They had to do *something* because my life and the life of our unborn baby was in the balance.

To complicate matters, Townsville hospital's birthing suite had been relocated to a building about 12km away from the main hospital. All birthing equipment had to be brought by ambulance immediately to the main hospital. The lumbar puncture results were not yet available, but my worsening severe symptoms pointed towards a case of herpes simplex viral encephalitis. Something had to be done immediately, so by 3am I was ready for transfer to Townsville General Hospital. It was a trip of about 5km. I was sedated, and intubated, with a paramedic squeezing a balloon to help me breathe. Roland was distraught. Pete had arrived at the hospital and met us as I was being wheeled out to the ambulance. He grabbed Roland around the shoulders and said, 'Go with the ambulance. I'll meet you at the General.'

At 3.10am I arrived at the hospital, and the orderly who collected me was Paul, a family friend of Roland's. Paul said that he would look after me, and he wheeled me off to intensive care in preparation for surgery. The nursing staff set me up on their machines while Roland and Pete were in the waiting room. Knowing that time was important, they were both allowed in to see me. They were told again that there was no other choice but to deliver the baby by emergency caesarean and then place me into a coma. They were warned that the baby may need resuscitation after delivery. Roland and Pete were then asked to return to the waiting room because staff had to get me to theatre.

Paul the orderly came back to see how Roland was doing. He asked if he would like him to ring Roland's parents (whom Paul had always called 'aunty' and 'uncle') to see if they would come to the hospital. Roland thanked Paul and asked if he could have only his dad (Pa) come up. In no time at all, Pa arrived and they all sat together waiting. Roland turned to his dad and said, 'If something happens to Sandra, I'm off. I just couldn't live here with so many memories. I'll get myself lost somewhere.' Pa replied, 'What about your boys?' Roland broke down and cried because he hadn't thought about his loved boys – he had been so worried about me. Then there was movement and they looked up to see two nurses pushing a humidicrib (an incubator for newborns), and ambulance personnel arriving, with them all going through to surgery. They were getting ready for the baby. It was happening.

There were eight doctors in attendance and they headed to Theatre 7 with Dr S. The anaesthetics were administered at 4.30am, the operation began at 4.45am and my baby boy was born at

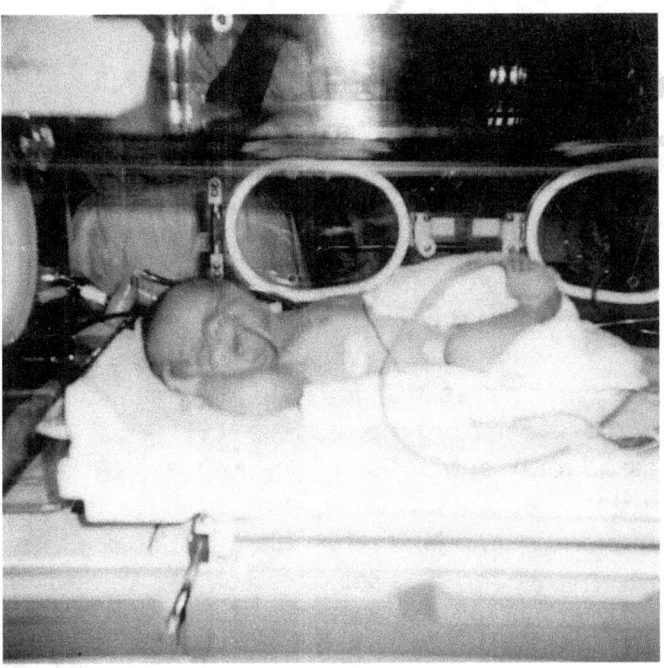

Precious Jaiden, just after he came into the world on 6 August 1994

4.49am, weighing 6lb 14oz. The operation completed at 5.10am and I was transferred to my room at 5.30am. It was all so quick and so efficient in order to save two lives. A nurse came out to the waiting room with the news – it was a boy and he was pink (so he hadn't needed resuscitation). There were many quiet tears of relief at that moment.

Needing to break the silence, Roland stood and announced the name of his newly born son to everyone: 'We have a son. His name is Jaiden Alexander.' This was the name we had chosen together. Our first son's middle name is Roland (after his dad), so for our third son we chose Alexander as the middle name because it is the masculine form of Sandra. Jaiden had been born and he was alive. About 10 minutes later the nurse brought Jaiden out to the waiting room, in his humidicrib. She handed him to Roland for that first cuddle, that oh-so-special cuddle. He was a perfect looking little boy. Roland handed him back to the nurse and asked for Pa to be allowed to visit Jaiden. Our baby was then placed back into the humidicrib and taken by ambulance to the women's hospital. He would go to the neonatal ward for two days of intensive care, followed by 12 days of special care. He would also be treated with the same drugs that I was receiving, just in case. We were told later that, luckily, my womb had protected Jaiden from the virus.

Dr R asked for IV antibiotics; IV acyclovir; an MRI; and an anaesthetic infusion that would induce the coma. Roland was allowed to sit and hold my hand while the nurses settled me into my room, attended to my wound and set up all of the IVs and machines. I didn't have the chance to hold my son or even to know that he had been born. I had been unconscious ever since they had sedated me before the transfer to the general hospital – and I was now to be placed into a coma.

Chapter 5

At about 9.30am Roland went out to phone everyone. My mum was arriving at 2pm and because she was on the plane when Jaiden was born, she had had no idea that he had come into the world. When mum changed planes in Brisbane, my sister Joanne was at the airport, ready to give her a big hug and tell her the good news that she had a new grandson and the not-so-good news that I had been placed into a coma.

When mum (Nanna) arrived in Townsville, she joined Roland, his parents and our boys to visit Jaiden. At the hospital they scrubbed up and donned masks and coats to see the most gorgeous little boy who had so many tubes attached. Nanna put both hands through the crib holes to touch him and said, 'I wish with all my heart it was your mummy touching you.' She told him all about his mummy and how she would be able to cuddle him soon. She said, 'Until then, Nanna will visit you twice a day and give you mummy love and nanna love.'

Our boys, Tyrnan and Kyle (aged nine and seven), looked over at their new little brother and started crying. They said they loved him but he looked so small and helpless. Having a baby brother wasn't happening in the way that I had told them it would and they were trying to understand it all. However, Jaiden was a little piece of happiness when everything looked so gloomy.

My dad had never coped with we kids being hurt so you can imagine that he would struggle with me being ill. So, when Roland rang my dad, he bluntly said to him, 'If you want to see your daughter alive, you need to get here now!' This, and encouragement from his lovely partner Jan, made him ring his nephew Ian, who owned planes for his freight delivery business. Ian said, 'Of course, Uncle Brian. I'll fly you up.' Ian loved teasing my dad with the 'uncle' label because Ian is only five years younger than him. We have all enjoyed many wonderful times together. When Ian and Dad arrived about three days later, Roland took the boys to meet Granddad at the airport. They went out onto the tarmac and hopped into the plane, sitting in the pilot's seat and pretending they were real pilots. The joys of the little things ... With so much happening, it was a much-needed distraction. Thank you, Ian.

Back in intensive care, my MRI results showed an extensive area of damage to the right temporal lobe. These findings were consistent with a herpes infection. The doctors knew that I now faced the fight of my life. If I survived, I could be paralysed down my left side and need 24/7 care.

My temperature would not come down, which indicated that the virus was still attacking me. With few options left, Dr R told Roland that he was going to triple my dose of medication. Roland asked Dr R what my chances were. Dr R said he didn't know – probably under 1%. He then looked at Roland and said, 'It's up to Sandra now.' All they could do was wait. I lay on that bed unaware of anything that was happening. I have the hospital and medical reports from that time, and these serve as a form of memory, as do photos and diary notes from family. They say that people may be able to hear when they are in a coma – I don't recall whether or not I did, but perhaps I did because I fought on.

Roland sat beside me, holding my hand and telling me everything I had to live for. He told me about our lives, including all the things we had done together and the places we had been. He wished for me to fight to stay here with him and the boys. Roland prayed, and pleaded with God: 'Please give her back to me, any way you can.' He didn't know how bad my brain injury would be if I did wake, but he knew that, whatever the outcome, he loved me and was going to take me home. Home to be with him and our boys.

Roland told Dr R point blank that I was not going into a care home. I had a home and I was going home with him. He would

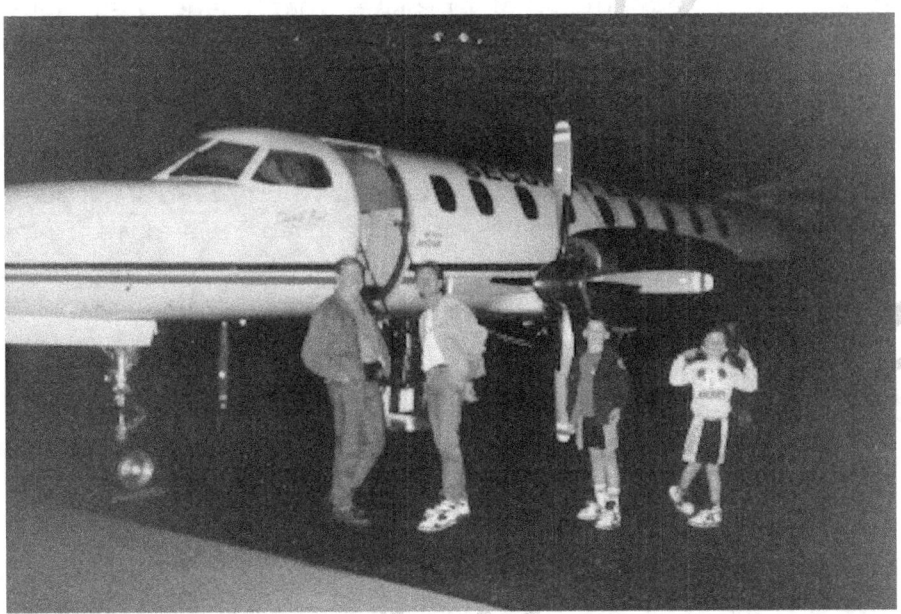
Brian (Dad), Roland, Tyrnan and Kyle

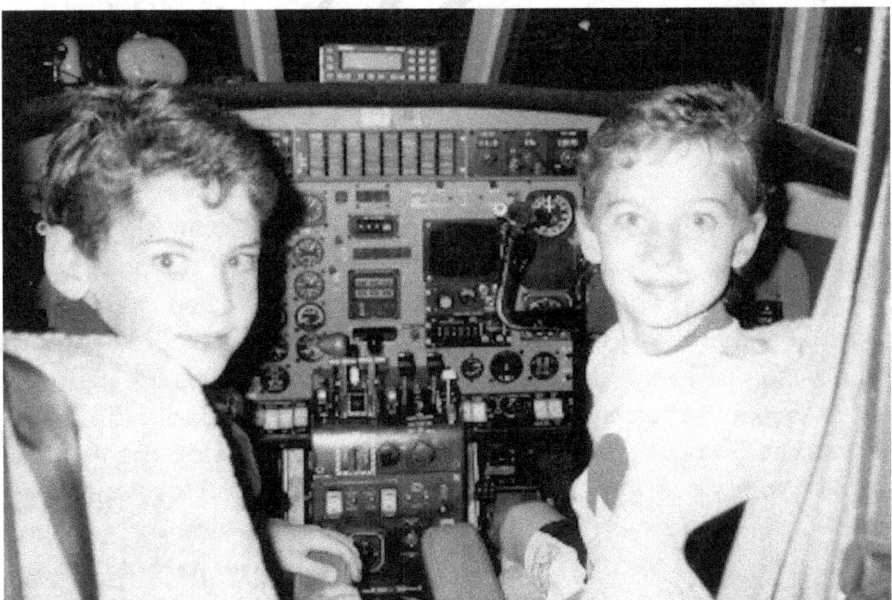
Co-pilots Tyrnan and Kyle

look after me, no matter what. Dr R knew that Roland was serious, so he handed him a piece of paper that listed his home and work phone numbers. He told Roland to ring him at any time if he needed anything.

Our dear friends and family sat outside intensive care with food and support for Roland. My mum came to visit me, and she placed her face next to mine to tell me that she loved me and was there for me. Then, Roland and Mum brought our boys up to see me. It was hard for them. Tyrnan couldn't touch me, and he choked up as he said, 'I love you, Mummy.' Kyle stroked my hair and also told me he loved me. They both talked close to my ear, hoping I could hear them. When it was time for them to leave, they said their prayers and asked Jesus to make Mummy well. That night Nanna placed her arms around her grandsons as they went to sleep, cuddled together.

It was during this time that I left my body on Earth. I left behind a body hooked up to machines that were keeping it alive. I felt that I was held by God, curled up on his lap with his arms around me. He soothed me and told me that I was safe. I felt the comfort, the warmth, the love ... and no pain. It was peaceful and tranquil, just like walking along the beach on a beautiful day. All you hear is the sound of waves breaking on the beach, your feet taking steps in the sand, and your breath going in and out. I felt my strength returning. I was then given a choice – I could stay there or I could go back.

All of a sudden I found myself sitting cross-legged above the doorway of my house. There was no roof, and I was watching Roland and my children. Roland was running from room to room trying to do everything and our boys were crying. I could see that Roland wasn't coping and I just wanted to be with them and comfort them all. My life was in that home with my family and it was breaking my heart to watch their distress. So, I turned to God and told him that I wanted to go back. There was nothing that would stop me from returning to my beautiful family. Making that decision was easier than my recovery was going to be, but I wasn't going to give up. I chose to come back and I fought harder to live than I've ever fought before.

Roland would visit me at the hospital every morning and say, 'Hi, honey, it's me,' and give me kiss. He would then hold my hand and stay all day. The nurses and doctors told him to talk to me because I

> *It was during this time that I left my body on Earth.*

could hear him. I don't recall what he said, but I do remember hearing male voices. The doctors said that my memories of that time are in my brain, but because of the drugs I was taking the memories would not have been stored in the correct way. I remember Roland holding my hand, and I could feel the warmth and love. I didn't feel alone. I simply had to come back.

My family visited and talked to me, giving me love and encouragement. My dad sat beside me, his beautiful daughter, for whom he couldn't do anything than 'be there'. He would rather be helping me to fix my motorbike or be running beside me just like when I was little, showing me how to let out the clutch on my bike. We had spent many hours together and even worked together and now all he could do was sit with me. He couldn't fix this situation.

I always had someone with me, and the nurses in intensive care were angels. They looked after me so well, including washing and braiding my hair and keeping me clean and respectable. However, I do recall feeling cold and the sheets being stiff. I was told later that because I had tubes going into me (including one directly into my heart, just in case it was needed for a dose of adrenalin), I was naked under those sheets. Whenever I think of cold hard sheets now it makes me smile because it proves that I did recall something of my time in intensive care. I have only soft sheets now.

The doctors knew that I needed a feeling of connection to life, so they made sure that I bonded with my newborn son. My wish had been to breastfeed, so the wonderful nurses made that happen. Every day an ambulance and nurse brought my little boy from the other hospital to visit me. He would be placed on my chest and the nurses would ensure that he received a breastfeed. They also expressed my milk and noted how much I was producing. It wasn't enough for a full feed, but I'm so thankful that my baby received some of his sustenance from me.

We have a large circle of very dear friends and our door had always been open for them. Prior to my ending up in hospital, every Wednesday night our friends Chris and Robert, and our nephew Jason, came over for dinner and to watch the TV series *The X-Files*. I loved being like a sister to our friends – they all felt like family. I especially felt this way about Robert, who was like the little brother I had always wanted. Robert's dad (John) and Roland had worked

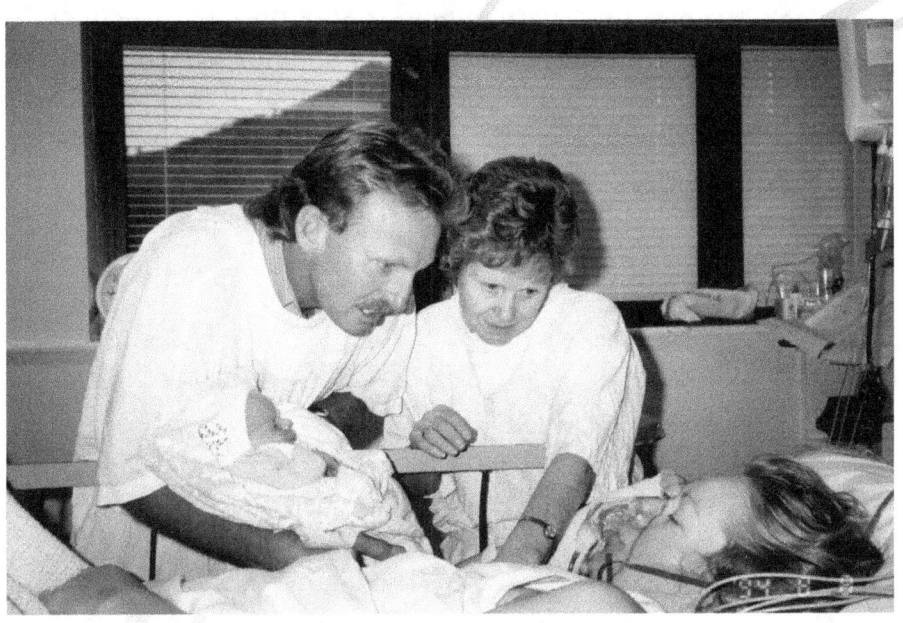
Being introduced to baby Jaiden while I was in the coma

together and now John's entire family had become part of our family. Robert treated our sons like they were his little brothers and drove them to karate and played games with them. They certainly needed that big brother now.

Our friends were all repaying our love by visiting me in hospital and by providing food and support to Roland (including looking after our children). Visitors were allowed in one at a time, with Roland, who had made the decision not to bring the boys back up to the hospital – it had just been so hard for them the first time. Our dear mate Pete would massage my feet when he visited me, not knowing what else to do. Little did he realise that this was the best way to stimulate my brain because nerve endings (which are found in the feet) send messages to the brain. Oh, that little foot massage treat stopped when I left hospital, but it's something we laughed about later!

Chapter 6

One afternoon nursing staff came in to check my caesarean wound. My mum was sitting beside me. As the nurse pushed on my stomach, I groaned and attempted to sit up. Mum said the nurse got the shock of her life because I shouldn't have been able to feel anything – I was in a coma! Mum smiled because she knew that I was there somewhere, trying to come back. The nurse quickly recovered and checked my medication, and the dosage was increased.

Every day there were more flowers, phone calls and best wishes. The company I worked for sent flowers from each of my three branches, as well as from the Brisbane office and the Melbourne head office. I also received flowers from some of the work suppliers with whom I dealt directly. Roland's workplace sent flowers and a teddy (which became Jaiden's favourite). My beautiful mum kept a record of the hundreds of people and companies who sent messages, cards, flowers and gifts so that when I woke up, I'd know how much I had been thought of. She noted if people sent get-well wishes or birth wishes, and if they visited me in hospital and took photos. Mum wanted to help me to fill in the gaps of those few weeks of my life. Thank you, Mum.

Not only were good wishes being sent to me – my name was also mentioned at many church services, where prayers were asked for me. So many people (many I didn't know) were praying for my survival and my health. I couldn't let them down, could I?! In my mind I must have summoned my strength and my courage. I must have taken a deep breath, placed my hands on my hips and said with determination, 'I'll do it myself.'

Dr R made the decision to reduce my sedation and continue with observations. He wanted to see what I was able to do after waking from the coma. After 10 days in the coma, with no one knowing the outcome during that time, the fog in my brain began to lift. I started to wake up faster than expected, opening my eyes and breathing spontaneously. I generally didn't respond to verbal commands but I would nod in response to simple, clear questioning. My eyes were opening more but I was drowsy. The doctors were happy that my pupils were reacting equally but they noticed that I was neglecting my left side so a physiotherapist was sent in to work with me. Tests were done, with the results documented as *'right side normal, left leg weakness, left arm severe weakness, smiles, obeys commands, no verbal responses at present'*.

At this time, I recall seeing nurses come into my room but I only remember seeing the bottoms of their dresses, and also seeing their hands when they placed a container on me before giving me an injection. They injected me twice a day to try to prevent stomach ulcerations that could occur because of the strong medication I was taking. I remember that the injections hurt. I also remember rubbing my lower tummy and feeling something odd there. My brain tried to work out what I was feeling because I couldn't sit up to see for myself. A nurse saw me and said, 'They are staples. We are taking them out this afternoon.' This made no sense to me. Staples? How did they get there and why were they there? I had no words to ask the nurse and I faded back to sleep.

I was becoming more alert, and a doctor asked me if I knew who he was. I replied, 'Yes, a doctor,' which was a very logical answer because he was wearing a doctor's outfit. He pointed to a nurse and I said, 'Nurse.' This, too, was logical because she was wearing a uniform. The doctor then pointed to Roland and asked who he was. I stared at Roland but I didn't have any idea as to who he was. He wasn't dressed like a doctor or a nurse. The question confused me because it was totally out of context. The doctor explained that this man was Roland, my husband. I was confused. We had been talking about doctors and nurses. Where did Roland fit in? I really didn't know who he was.

CHAPTER 6

Roland was heartbroken because he thought he had lost me again. Seeing this, the doctor stopped asking questions and explained to Roland that this could be temporary and that he should give it time. I was very confused and looked around, staring at the flowers, cards and photos in my room. It was as though I hadn't seen flowers of those types and colours before. I had woken up in unfamiliar surroundings and everything looked foreign. I couldn't really comprehend where I was or why I was there. What was the thing that was attached to me? What did it do? Who was I?

Roland was eager for any sign that I knew him. However, it was hard for me to sort out my thoughts because the drugs I had been taking were so strong (my family had even been able to smell them). I was sent for another MRI to check whether or not I'd had any further seizures while I was in the coma. I was also moved to another ward. I was very confused with myself and didn't feel connected to anything or anyone. Roland was always there, and this made me feel relaxed and protected although I didn't know why. I kept looking at his hands. They must have been important to me. One evening Roland wanted to feed me, and in doing so he spilled a little on my chin and clothes. But when he went to clean me up, the nurses said not to worry about it; they would do it. Roland kissed me goodnight and left.

At 6am the next day, Roland came to see me and greeted me with, 'Hi, honey, it's me,' and a kiss. However, when he saw the food still on my chin and my clothes, he went berserk. He started yelling at the nurses. At that moment Dr R walked in and saw what had happened. He quietly asked Roland to stop, and to go to get a drink. He said that he would handle it. Roland had a lot of respect for, and trust in, this doctor, so he nodded and did as he was asked. When Roland returned to my room, he found me showered, cleaned and ready for transfer to another ward, where I would have my own room. Dr R wanted the best of care for me so he had me moved to another area of the hospital.

The hospital was having renovations done, and on the way to my new room they wheeled me past some workmen. To my delight, I saw a familiar face of our dear mate, Chris. Wow! I recognised someone and knew his name! We said a quick hello and cheeky Chris wished me well as they pushed me to my new room.

> *I was very confused and looked around, staring at the flowers, cards and photos in my room.*

CHAPTER 6

Nobody knew what deficiencies I would have as a result of my massive brain injury. My speech was quiet and slow, and I was slow to understand and obey commands. I needed help to shower and it was decided that I should have no visitors during meals because it was too distracting – I'd concentrate on the conversation instead of eating (I was still not feeding myself, either). Since waking from the coma, I had complained about a noise in my left ear. However, nobody seemed to be doing anything about it and it was getting worse. I was unsteady on my feet, with my brain feeling as though it was a mass of water moving in my head. This made me feel totally unbalanced. I often felt confused and as though I couldn't connect with anything. I knew that I had a baby son but I don't remember the moment I was told. Looking back later, I remembered the excitement I had felt at the birth of our first two sons, but this time it had felt empty. Everything felt strange and weird. Dr R noted that I also showed signs of depression.

In the meantime, my mum was getting my house in order so that it would be running smoothly when Jaiden and I came home. The boys were finding it hard not having me home, and Mum initiated a routine that helped to make things feel normal: clean the house, keep the washing up to date, walk the boys to school, go to the Kirwan hospital to see Jaiden, head back to pick up the boys from school, go back to the Kirwan hospital to see Jaiden, and then go to the hospital to see me.

When my sister Joanne came for a visit, I knew who she was as soon as she walked into the room. This was my awesome big sister who I felt would make all of these bad things go away ... just as she had when I was five years of age. It was at that age that I had fallen and broken my leg – she had picked me up and carried me to our parents. All of those memories were there for me and I felt safe again.

Taking your baby home is a special time, and I missed that precious moment with Jaiden. Before my brain injury, I had been looking forward to it, and now I can only look at photos that were taken for me. Roland made bringing Jaiden home into a family event. Along with my awesome sister, our boys and Nanna, Roland went to the Kirwan hospital on 20 August to pick up our 14-day-old son. They then drove straight up to me so that we could all be together for the first time in two weeks. I was propped up in bed with

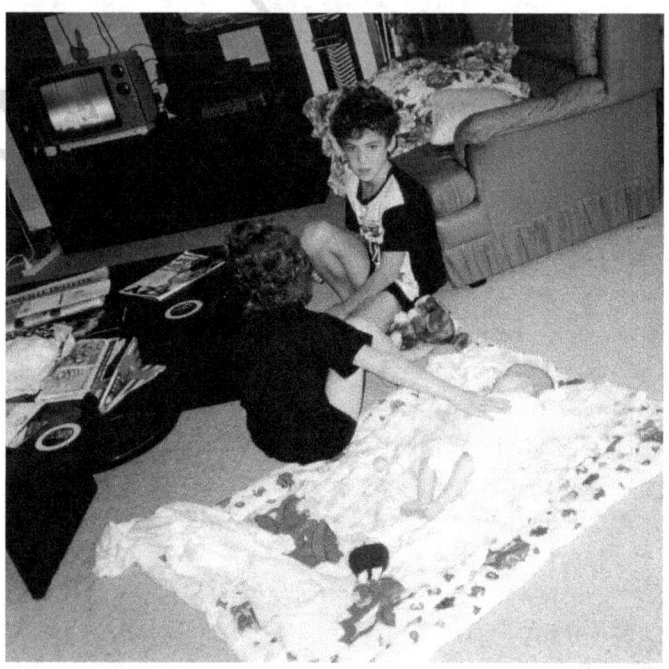

Tyrnan and Kyle doting on their baby brother

CHAPTER 6

my IV lines, but I was able to hug my family and feel part of it (even if I couldn't go home with them afterwards). To the boys, I may have looked like Mummy but I seemed different, so they were very careful and quiet around me.

My family took turns visiting us and had to travel long distances to reach us. There was always a family member staying at our home to help Roland with our two sons and our newborn. Mum said that Jaiden was a dear little boy and so good. The boys loved feeding their brother. Nanna settled into a new routine of putting washing on the line, taking the boys to school, and then heading off to the hospital with Jaiden, to see me. Mum said that it was so hard when I asked her to leave Jaiden with me at the end of each visit. It was incredibly difficult for her to walk out that door and leave me behind. I was bonding with my son and wanted him with me. Those motherly feelings were coming back.

At home, Roland wanted to do it all himself, and my mum gave him space. Roland worked all day, visited me, and wanted to look after his youngest son at night. Once the night feed was done, he watched a movie to help him unwind. Then, because the next feed was only a couple of hours away, he watched another movie. He did this for a couple of nights. Deprived of sleep, on the third night he slept through and woke in the morning saying, 'Oh, wow, Jaiden slept through last night!' Mum smiled and told him that she woke to the sounds of the crying baby. She got up and fed Jaiden, leaving Roland to sleep. He was so tired, and sleeping through the noise of a crying baby made him realise that he couldn't do it alone and needed to take turns with Mum for the night feeds.

I was hooked up to an IV of acyclovir, and to allow me to be mobile, the IV machine was on wheels – it had to go everywhere with me, and I named it 'Harry'. Whenever I walked unsteadily to the toilet, Harry came with me. This walk was a feat in itself because I had little to no short-term memory. To walk to the toilet, I would ask for directions from my husband, or from a family member or friend who was with me. I would then walk down the corridor in the right direction, get to the nurses' desk, and ask for someone to point to where the toilet was. From there, I would check every room until I found the toilet. Upon leaving the toilet I would walk back to the nurses' desk, and a nurse would point the way to my room. I would look in every room until I found my room. My room always had heaps of flowers and photos on display. Sometimes the journey back was quicker because I'd look up and see Roland or Pete spying on me and I would confidently walk to them.

I was so frustrated by the difficulties of that journey because I knew that it shouldn't be as hard as it was to remember the way. I wanted to be able to walk there and back myself. As a solution, I asked Roland to bring me stickers. 'Why stickers?' he asked. I told him that I was going to stick them on the floor so that I could get to the toilet and back without having to ask anyone for directions. I was very determined and I knew that I couldn't get lost if I followed the stickers. My logical thinking and independence were surfacing. No, Roland didn't bring stickers, and the nurses said that for health and safety reasons they wouldn't have let me stick them on the floor anyway. This was a pity because stickers really would have helped.

When Pete and Roland visited me one evening, I yet again asked where the toilet was. This time they played a joke on me and pointed in the opposite direction. I had a feeling that it was the wrong direction but my stubborn nature was too great, and off I went with Harry the IV machine. I looked in every room until I eventually found a different toilet. I wasn't going to let them win. They had begun to get worried that they had done the wrong thing. I found my way back, feeling happy that I had outsmarted them. I was that determined little girl who had her hands on her hips, saying, 'I'll find it myself.'

I was having regular blood tests and other tests to check on my progress. Between all of the tubes that had been down my throat, a catheter, a direct adrenaline line and IVs, I was a little 'over' all of the pain. My arms were black and blue from needles. (I still rub my forearms at the memory of this.) I continued to complain often about the noise in my left ear, but my complaints seemed to fall on deaf ears. For simple tasks like sitting up, lifting my arm or sitting on the toilet, the nurses would have to explain, step by step, how to do these things – or I would just stare at the nurses, looking bewildered. One day I was rubbing at my IV site and a nurse asked me what I was doing. I replied, 'Just trying to decide what to do with this.' I smile as I type this because I realise now that my brain was trying to work out what the IV site was and what I could do with it. I did remove a couple of IVs – but in my defence, nobody told me not to!

I started to become defensive about my baby and was determined to feed him myself. Dr R saw that my memory was getting

CHAPTER 6

better and that I was speaking more. I'd read the nametags of the nurses and say their names. I had facial recognition issues so I couldn't recognise who was whom; however, I could read and remember names. I recall receiving a phone call from the work colleague who was doing my job. We chatted about work and about balancing the sales tax account. Work mode stepped in and I really wanted to go straight to work to sort it out. Yet when this colleague asked me which hospital room I was in so that he could visit me, I had no idea and had to let Roland talk with him.

So, after three weeks in hospital, it was decided that we would work towards me being able to go home. Home to be with my husband, who would help me with anything I needed. It would take another week before we got the all-clear. Roland made sure family would be available to stay with us. My mum and our sons were waiting at home for me.

However, a social worker visited us in hospital and carefully explained to Roland that it would be difficult to care for me at home because I wasn't able to care for myself. We were told that 95% of marriages fail when the husband becomes the main carer. This is because the man is usually ill-equipped to provide the level of care that the woman needs. I could recognise my natural family but I had to be told who Roland and the boys were. Roland gave her the same answer that he had given everyone else: 'Sandra is my wife and she will be coming home with me – and I can look after her.'

Roland had promised God that he would have me back in any way that he could, and he wasn't going back on his promise. Yes, I became very disorientated and had little to no short-term memory. Yes, I needed help to shower and get dressed. Yes, I needed prompting to do things. Yes, I needed clear instructions. However, I was able to do things such as eat a meal by myself. There were probably many more things that we would have to cope with but we would face all of that together. I was his wife, he loved me and he was taking me home.

The nurses knew I was ready to go home when a male nurse asked if it would be OK for him to help me shower. 'What, a male?!' my brain said. I realised for the first time that the nurse was male and I stood up, put my hands on my hips, said, 'No, I'll do it myself.' He smiled because he realised that I was getting better. Dr R

> *Roland had promised God that he would have me back in any way that he could, and he wasn't going back on his promise.*

CHAPTER 6

then reviewed me for the last time in hospital. He decided that I was ready to go home.

With many obstacles in front of us and with Roland holding my arm, we walked slowly to the car. This was the start of our new journey together. At that moment I may not really have remembered the man who was walking beside me, but I felt safe and loved. I had said to my mum that Roland must be really special or I wouldn't have married him. So, I would have to get to know him all over again.

My steps to the car were sluggish and it took all of my effort. I felt the weight of the world on my shoulders, but I was going home. At that time, 'home' was just a word, but I felt as though it would be my safe place and that I would get better there. While I was in the coma, the doctors had thought I wouldn't be able to walk unassisted when I woke – balance was expected to be an issue because the area of the brain that controls it was very damaged – and yet there I was. I looked forward to proving the doctors wrong in many other areas, too. I took one step at a time as I made my way towards the car, and I took a deep breath as I got inside. The car felt a bit claustrophobic (it was much smaller than the room I was used to in hospital) and the roof felt so close to my head. On the journey home I had to ask Roland to slow down because everything was going past so quickly. It was like being on a rollercoaster without holding on. I wanted to close my eyes but that wouldn't have helped me avoid feeling the movement of the car and sensing the shadows as we passed buildings and trees.

I was happy to be going home but everything along the journey looked new and foreign and we were moving too fast for me to take it all in – it was overwhelming. I would notice a tree and start drawing it in my mind, analysing it and searching for it in my memory. In the meantime, we had sped past the tree and my mind would have to move on. I felt very anxious, like a small lost child. When I reflect on it now, I am reminded of the mud races Roland and I took part in all those years ago. On this trip it was Roland giving *me* directions. He was telling me which way we were going, and all the while he was holding my hand. Our journey was taking us home, and my recovery was about to begin.

Chapter 7

Although I recall the drive from the hospital, I have no memory of arriving home on Saturday 27 August 1994. We pulled up on the paved driveway that we had built, a driveway leading up to our home of five years. This was the home for which I had helped Roland add a brick veneer. There was the awesome fancy brick letterbox, and a path with the three steps Roland had made for me up to the patio. It should have been two steps but I had always dreamed of three steps that featured side walls – like a big grand staircase – with pot plants sitting on the tops of the walls. Roland made that happen for me. We had planted and worked so hard together to make our dreams come true, but now I didn't recognise any of it.

The boys heard the car pull up and went crazy with excitement inside because their mummy was home. They raced to me to give me cuddles as we walked in the door. I flinched at first because of the noise and the movement, and then I hugged them. I felt confused about my surroundings. It was as though I had been picked up and shaken around. Nothing looked familiar as I walked into the loungeroom. I had made all of the curtains and we had painted the walls together. But, to me, it looked like someone else's home. Mum was sitting on the lounge, giving me time to take it all in, and that's when I saw it – the photo. The wedding photo on the wall. The lady in the wedding dress was me and the man standing beside me was Roland. Logically, my mind said, 'It must be true. Roland is my husband.' I found it hard to take my eyes off of the photo, and I wished that all my memories would come back.

Have you ever woken in the middle of the night and wondered where you were and what was happening? That was me, in the middle of the day in my own home.

Seeing my distress, Roland took my hand and said, 'Come on. Let's show you around the house.' As we walked into the dining room I noticed the brick feature wall, and it felt comforting but I didn't know why. We headed through to the kitchen and I looked out the window into our yard. I was still trying to understand what was going on and what to feel.

We only had a small, three-bedroom, one-bathroom home but nothing looked familiar. I made sure I held onto Roland's hand for support because I was feeling unsteady on my feet. I could feel my brain moving like a wave in my head, just as it had done in hospital. The wave flowed down my spine, and it felt so weird. The sensation frightened me and I waited for it to pass. Walking up the hallway, it felt as though I stepped into a hole and I nearly fell over. My balance was all over the place, just like walking on a boat. Roland caught me and with a smile said, 'Oh, I've still got it. You looked at me and the earth moved.' This was the moment that I needed. It felt magical as we both smiled and hugged. For the first time in weeks, and for that brief moment, I felt normal, I felt loved and I felt safe.

We walked into the baby's nursery and I gazed around, trying to connect with the motherly feelings I knew I should have. Our sleeping baby was in his bassinette, the same one his brothers and his mummy had slept in. I gently touched his skin and felt his warmth. A small smile appeared on my face as I remembered that this was my son. We left quietly to let him sleep.

As we walked into the boys' shared room, I could hear my mum talking to them in the loungeroom. 'It's OK, Mummy isn't well, so let's give her some space and time. Mummy loves you.' My heart broke because I didn't know how to fix this situation and make their mummy better.

As we walked towards our bedroom, there was so much to take in. I looked up and had a flash of a memory of sitting above the doorway but that didn't make any sense to me. Nothing was making sense. Roland opened my wardrobe and I stared inside it, trying to understand what all of the items were. He told me that they were my clothes and my shoes. I didn't understand what that meant so I

CHAPTER 7

held out my hand and started to feel their texture. My clothes. Feeling very confused, I thought to myself, 'So what do I do with them?'

Roland could see that it was all too much for me to take in, so he said we'd go back to the loungeroom where we could sit and relax. I really just wanted to curl up in a ball and make all of this confusion stop but I didn't want to let go of Roland's hand. He was my lifeline.

I found it hard to relax because the boys wanted to sit with me and chatter. I was very sensitive to sound and movement, so I sat there, bewildered. Our boys – who had been so excited to have Mummy home – were now confused. I looked like Mummy but I didn't act or sound like Mummy. So, they didn't know how to behave around me.

Mum put on a movie to help distract them for a while. The movement on the television was too much for me, so I stared around the room. I then stared up at our wedding photo, hoping that I would feel some connection. Here I was, finally at my home, but it didn't feel like my home.

I stared down at my forearms. They looked weird because they featured bruises from my wrists to my elbows in varying shades of yellow, green, black and purple. These were from all of the drips and injections in hospital. I kept rubbing my forearms as if to try to soothe them or to remove the bruises. I knew that there was pain attached to these bruises. Mum watched me, and without a word stood up and left the room. In a moment she was back with a small jewellery box and she sat down beside me.

She opened the box and showed me my precious rings. Mum knew that these rings, and the love from those who had given them, meant the world to me. In hospital Roland had had to remove them from my fingers and had given them to my mum for safekeeping. They were all special and had different memories attached to them. My eternity ring was very special because it had been a complete surprise to receive it a few days before our fourth wedding anniversary. Roland had asked our dear friend Craig to make it for me. One night Craig had looked at my engagement ring and commented that a few of the claws needed to be fixed. He had often done this sort of repair work for me over the years so I didn't think anything of it. I gave him the ring, knowing that I'd have it back within a couple of days. Little did I know that Craig needed my engagement ring so that he could design and make my eternity ring to match it. Combined with my wedding ring, it would make a lovely set. Roland couldn't keep the secret for long and gave it to me early. Seeing those rings brought back the beautiful, loving memories of that time, and made me feel more like myself.

The three other rings in the box were given to me by the most precious ladies I had known, loved and adored. The first was the wedding ring from my grandma (Mum's mum), which she had given me on my wedding day as my 'something old' – she wore her husband's (my Poppa's) ring instead of her own. The second was the eternity ring from my dear nan (Dad's mum). The third ring was the wedding band of my awesome great-grandma (Poppa's mum). I had always worn these rings because they made me feel loved, and they reminded me of wonderful times spent together.

I looked down at the rings on my fingers and enclosed my hands around them. I now had something to focus on. Something to stir comforting feelings from my childhood. The heirloom rings brought back lovely memories such as standing beside my great-grandma in her kitchen, with me turning the handle to make butter. I also remembered standing with Poppa beside my great-grandma's hospital bed after she had had a stroke. If nothing else, the rings made me know and feel that I was loved.

Everyone seemed to be tiptoeing around me, so it was important to get into a routine that gave us all a sense of normality. To start us off, we sat down together at the table for the lunch that mum had made us. With an eerie quiet we slowly ate our lunch, not wanting to look up or talk. Everyone was probably thinking, 'What do we do now?' For me it was, 'Who am I?'

Chapter 8

Nobody had explained to us what to expect or do when we got home. Mum and Roland would find out what I could and couldn't do. They would then fill in the gaps and try to make our home life as normal as possible. I didn't really recall how to run a household, or everyday things such as what seat I should sit in at mealtimes. I needed clear instructions. Questions to me had to be clearly worded and asked one at a time. My speech was slow and I needed to be given time to reply to each question. My mind went blank often and it was hard for me to make any decisions.

My left hand would shake and I would stare at it, wondering what it was doing. Two days after arriving home we were due for an appointment with Dr R, so we would have to wait until then to ask him all of our questions. I sat in our lounge chair and felt defeated, fully aware that everything wasn't OK. I had so looked forward to being able to come home. I had imagined that once I was home, somehow everything would be OK ... but it wasn't. Because I was very tired, Roland helped me walk to our room for a rest. Doctors had said that I would tire easily because my brain was still healing and because I was taking certain drugs.

Roland settled me into our bed. It felt so different and so much softer than the hospital beds (which had given me a sore back). We had a soft-sided, double-bladder waveless waterbed and it was so comfy. I tried to ignore my back pain and went to sleep, hoping that when I woke up everything would have been a dream and I'd be me again.

When I woke from my nap, I wondered where I was. Everything was so confusing. It's hard to lose over three weeks of your life and to have no real recollection of being sick, having fits or being in intensive care. I would have to learn to live with this situation and re-learn 'being me' every morning. I could hear people talking elsewhere in the house, so I felt determined to get up, walk down the hallway into the loungeroom and start to re-learn how to be me.

The rest of the first day back at home was spent sitting quietly in the lounge in a state of confusion, with my family looking after me. I noticed that when I needed to go to the toilet, I had to get there in a hurry. I wondered why that was. Mum told me that I was able to wait long periods before needing to go to the toilet. I analysed this, and over time worked out that I needed to go to the toilet in the morning when I woke. I would then need to go again about half an hour after a drink at breakfast or lunch. I was aware that a pattern was emerging, so I paid attention to how my body felt at these times. Over the next few weeks, I re-learned my body's responses to many stimuli and began to understand each difference.

Mum said that I became very protective of Jaiden and tried my best to look after him. I was still trying to breastfeed him but because I didn't have enough milk, everyone took turns to bottle-feed him after I had breastfed him. This meant that he had a full meal. The boys enjoyed feeding their brother. Feeding my son gave me a purpose and a job, and I tried to do all I could for my baby. However, Mum kept asking me why I hadn't changed Jaiden's nappy. She said it was very obvious from the smell that he had done a poo. After Mum said this, I would get up and change his nappy. I hadn't at all realised that he had done a poo. This nappy issue kept happening but nobody thought much about it. They just thought that my short-term memory was causing issues, and that I was having to cope with a lot.

When the first day at home was over, it was time for bed and a shower. Here I was 32 years of age, standing in the shower looking down at my body, water running down it, and having no idea where to start or what to do. I became so frustrated that I stared at the wall of the shower, as if I would get answers from it. I'm a logical thinker, so because the water ran down my body I thought that perhaps I should follow the water's direction to wash myself. The water hit my face first so I started there, followed by my neck, left arm, right

> *I became so frustrated that I stared at the wall of the shower, as if I would get answers from it.*

arm, front torso, back, left leg and foot, and then the right leg and foot. Going left then right, just like marching, made sense to me. OK, I did wash the left leg twice, but I had short-term memory issues and nobody was watching! It took a lot of effort to concentrate on showering so I knew that I had to make the process easier. I would think about it and work on it for next time.

Our first night together and I was back in our comfortable bed. However, I found it difficult to relax because so much had happened that day and I had had lots to take in. The lights were off and I hated being in the dark. It scared me – it reminded me of those nights alone in hospital and of being in a coma. Fear crept in and I felt panicky. Next to me I felt the warmth of Roland, so I curled up in his arms, where I felt safe. In the arms of my protector, I didn't have to remember anything, I didn't have to pretend to be OK and I didn't have to think. I could, for the first time in ages, be me. I closed my eyes and listened to Roland's heartbeat and to his breathing. The world had finally stopped moving. The rollercoaster ride was over for now and in that moment I felt like myself again.

We all need a safe place. In Roland's arms I was safe but I knew that I couldn't stay in his arms forever. I needed to stand up, face the world and find ways to cope. I had to re-learn everything and I had to find ways to learn and to remember. I was determined to be me again.

The first few weeks at home are a blur. Everyone worked around me and I mainly slept, or sat in the loungeroom trying my best to look after my baby. When we left the house, it was to visit doctors or to have blood tests. Our visit to Dr R had been helpful because he explained that my brain had to work twice as hard as everyone else's. This was why I would get tired easily. I had to give my brain time to heal and I'd stay on the prescribed medication for two years to make sure I had the best chance of recovery. Dr R didn't expect me to have any further seizures but he said that if I did, they would only be minor ones. I wouldn't be allowed to drive for a two-year period and I remember thinking 'drive'? Where would I drive? I got lost in my own home.

Dr R shared with us that he still couldn't believe that I had survived. He told us that I had aged him 10 years over the past month, and he reminded us that we could call him at any time, if needed. He was happy with my progress, he would arrange regular visits to keep

CHAPTER 8

an eye on my recovery, and I'd have further blood tests. When Dr R examined me, he noted that there was still weakness on my left side.

I was determined to get better but found the noise and movement at home very distracting. My left ear heard every noise all at once – people breathing, doors opening or closing, the clock ticking, sounds on the TV, children talking … even the sound of the breeze that was created when someone walked past me. It was as though someone had turned up the volume of my hearing to rock-concert level. If a pin had dropped onto a hard floor it would have sounded like a knife clanging onto the ground. Imagine your neighbour having a loud party and all you hear is the boom of the music and the murmur of people talking. This was what it was like for me, constantly. I couldn't block out the noise and it affected my concentration.

My vision was also an issue, with the walls and floor often looking like ripples on the ocean. Sometimes I could see little particles floating in the air, and I had what felt like tunnel vision. My balance wasn't good and I was scared that I would have another seizure.

I would ask what clothes I should wear, and I tried to do small jobs around the house. However, what could I do? Small household chores were difficult because I continually forgot to either do something or finish something. In my head, I had a picture of what I thought I should be able to do, but I didn't seem to be able to follow through on that vision. I couldn't remember how much soap to put in the washing machine or in the sink. However, I found that if I put things into a sequence, I could remember more: lid up on washing machine, pour in soap powder, put in clothes, shut lid, turn dial and press 'start'. I would sometimes forget what I had done so I would keep checking and re-checking. Every task took so long to do. Sometimes I also had to be reminded to take my medicine.

In the morning and after school, our boys would run to hug me and I'd experience a protective reflex movement where I would put up my hands and move my body back to push them away. The movement and noise of them running towards me hurt my head. This upset them because they thought it meant Mummy didn't love them. I did love them, but I also didn't understand why I was pushing them away and why it hurt my head.

I felt lost in my own little world and looked forward to Roland coming home every day. I often sat in the loungeroom staring at our wedding photo, using all my strength to summon memories. I had tried to watch TV but found that I couldn't remember what had happened in movies or shows, or who the people were. Everything moved too fast on the screen and I couldn't focus or take it all in. It became too difficult and I became very upset.

Seeing my distressed state, Roland started playing my favourite music to see if that would help. On hearing music by Phil Collins, my body started to respond straight away. I started to feel relaxed and began to sway with the music. Then I started to sing along softly to the songs. Wow! Another connection, and something that felt 'normal'. I couldn't remember where my bedroom was yet I could remember the words of these songs. This made me happy, and listening to Phil's music became my safe place. It helped settle my hearing, and it made me able to be in the moment, to feel real. It made such a difference to my day-to-day life, helping me remember a time when I was happy and healthy. It had triggered something in my brain and it felt good.

I was becoming more and more aware of my surroundings. In the loungeroom, I saw a bookcase full of books and was drawn to it. I had been a bookworm since I was a kid and always had a couple of books on the go at any time. I loved my library of books and had always remembered the stories in each one. Now, I held a book in my hand and wondered what it was and what I should do with it. It somehow felt familiar, so I opened it. As I gazed at the pages, the writing looked as though it was made up of jumbled-up letters. Nothing about them made sense, so I returned the book to the shelf.

Whenever I reached for something, I realised that my perspective of distance had been affected. I was very aware of trying to work out where my arms and legs were. It was if they were foreign to me. If I reached for something quickly, I would knock over the item or not reach it at all. Instead, I would stare at the object that I wanted and imagine my hand reaching for it. Brains are amazing – it felt as though a beam would go out from my eyes to the object (in the way that a tape measure does) and then return to my brain. I'm sure there must have been a small calculator in my head because I could almost feel my brain working out the distance and the angle. All of this took a couple of seconds, and I would then lift my hand and reach out for the item. Doing this made it easy to pick up and carry the item. I had accomplished something and, without realising it, I had reconnected one part of my brain to another.

> *... listening to Phil's music became my safe place.*

To help with my balance, I decided to start throwing a small ball from one hand to the other. I dropped it many times but eventually caught it. To add challenge, I moved my hands further apart, then closer, and then I threw the ball higher and lower. After this, I would close my eyes and do it all again. I kept doing this until I caught the ball almost all of the time. I had to make the right and left sides of my brain work together, and this exercise helped tremendously.

Over time, I didn't need to consciously calculate distances in my head – until I started driving, that is, because I would then have to re-learn how to cover certain distances at different speeds. We would discover later that all of my re-learning was creating new connections in my brain. However, in 1994 doctors and scientists were not aware that the brain was capable of this. They were under the impression that what you had, you lived with, and that brain cells didn't grow back. They were in for the surprise of their lives.

A week or two after I came home, Mum and I would walk the boys to school each day, and this helped to get me out of the house for exercise. It also felt good to be doing something normal and useful and to be included. The lollipop people (crossing guards) at school were happy to see me after hearing that I'd been ill.

One day, I approached a pile of envelopes that were sitting on our table. I wondered what the envelopes were so I picked up one and felt it. I turned it over, and something inside me triggered and made me automatically open it and unfold the piece of paper. I knew that that was what you did. I went ahead and opened them all. Then I looked at them and wondered what I should do with them. The best part about being left-brain strong is that I am analytical and logical. So, I started to sort the papers into ones that looked alike or that had dollar amounts on them. I re-sorted them when I realised that some had the same information at the top. The more I looked at them, the more information I saw. However, it became too confusing so I piled them up together for another day. They were, in fact, all of the invoices for my blood tests, along with reminders, statements from our private health cover, and receipts.

I would continually stare at our wedding photo and at Roland's hands in the photo. Hands … I kept focusing on hands. It was as if I wanted to feel those hands and remember the first time Roland held my hand. Roland had told me the story of how we had met and that I had made it difficult for him to hold my hand. All those

CHAPTER 8

years ago I had known that once I let Roland hold my hand, I could never take it back. We would be together forever. I wanted those memories back.

Feeling a strong need to put myself back together, I started to go through our photo albums. I learned all about my life. I recognised all my friends and family from the time of my birth to the 1980s. I felt as though I was an actress or an alien that knew all about a lady named Sandra Hubert, and that I had to act like her and make everyone believe it was Sandra.

When long-time friends came to visit, I would know who they were and I would chat with them, but as soon as they walked out the door, I forgot who had visited. During these visits I relied on my mum to make everything right and to help me work out what to say or do. Friends told me later that it was a case of me looking like the lights were on but nobody was home. That may sound cruel but it was the best analogy. That is how I looked. We laughed about it later and I know they were all very worried about me and also wanted to support Roland.

Chapter 9

Everything was an effort for me. However, as I've mentioned previously, I could work things out if I created systems. In the shower I lined up the bottles in order of use – face cleanser, body wash, shampoo and conditioner. I would lift the lid of the one I was going to use, and after I had used it, I would shut the lid and move on to the next bottle. With this easy system I didn't have to rely on my memory. Because it was so visual, I could remember it easily.

I also thought it would be good to write things down. This would help when I went to the doctor because I could refer to my list (and not my memory) to ask him all the things I wanted to know. However, it seemed that writing was a skill I had to re-learn. The first time I attempted it, I put my notepad on the table and sat down with a pen in my hand, ready to write. I had a slight tremor in my hands and this upset me because I didn't want them to shake. I stared at my shaking hands, and with all my strength tried to keep them from shaking. No, they wouldn't stop. Because I really wanted to write, I was determined to press on. I slowly formed the words in my head and tried to get them to flow to my hand. Guess what? Nothing happened.

I sat there with a pen – which was correctly held in my right hand – hovering over the paper. I stared at it. I just couldn't get my hand to move. It felt blocked and I didn't understand why. In frustration, I used my left hand to push the pen onto the paper and simultaneously used my feet to push my chair backwards. Looking down at the piece of paper, I saw that I had drawn a black line. I felt empowered. I took a deep few breaths and, with determination, started to move my right shoulder forwards and backwards, keeping my arm stiff and the pen on the paper. This created more lines. 'Good,' I thought. 'This is working.' Then I tried moving my wrist and elbow, and this made more black lines appear on the paper. The connection in my brain was made. In my mind, I started to form letters slowly to make the words that I wanted to write. It then became easy to physically write the words.

It was then I realised that I didn't remember how to spell. I had a memory of my dad and I sitting at a table and me asking him how to spell a word. I could hear my dad saying, 'Look it up in the dictionary.' (This was the same reply he had always given me when I asked how to spell a word!) I smiled at the memory and, just as I had done in the past, I pulled out that same dictionary and my trusty *Roget's Thesaurus*. Both books had been well used by me over the years and they were easy for me to read. Now I could look up the spellings of words and discover their meanings and I also felt satisfied because I had worked it out myself.

My goal was to read books again and to read the newspaper, just as I had done every morning since I was a young girl. My dad and I would have coffee together in the morning and read the paper, and then he would take me to school on a motorbike or in the car. Reading now took a lot of my energy and concentration, but I kept going. When writing there would be a delay between my thoughts and my hand. When I read back over my writing, I realised that often I started one word but finished it with the last letters of the following word. I'd look at the made-up word and wonder what I'd done. Sometimes I'd miss a word altogether. 'Take it slower,' I thought to myself. I knew that when I mastered writing I'd be able to write lists and notes to help re-train my memory.

It felt as though everything I needed to know was locked up somewhere in my brain. I just had to locate the key to open my brain and then store the information where I could find it again easily. Imagine a king was coming to visit you. How would you stand? What would you say? How would you act? I faced the same feeling of a lack of knowledge with everything I did – everything felt new to me.

It broke Roland's heart to see me struggle so much. He was very supportive but he couldn't fix these problems for me. Often, he

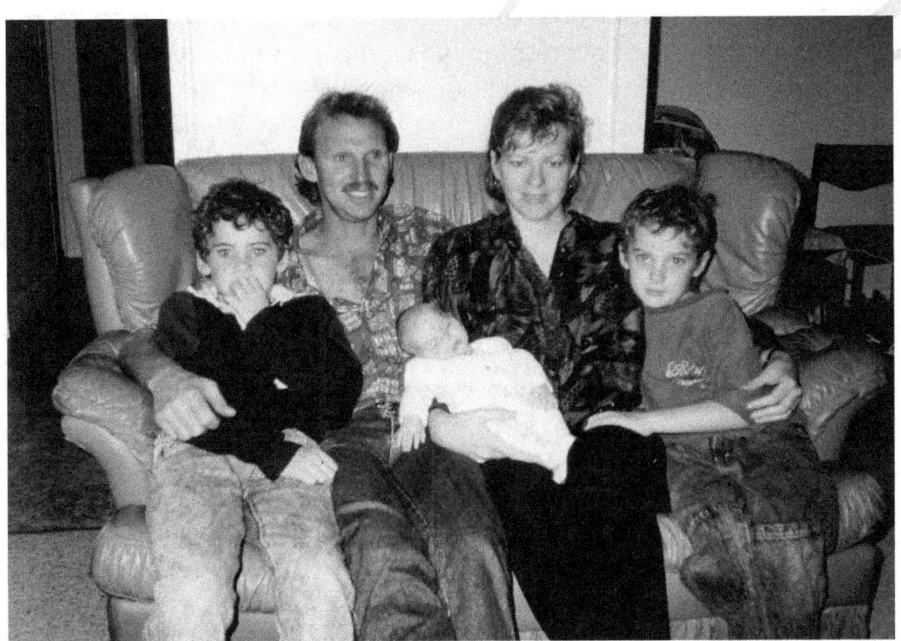

Jaiden at two months of age – we were all doing our best not to show our pain and confusion

couldn't stay to watch me, so to help him cope he'd go out to the shed and work on our four-wheel-drive off-road racing car.

I have always enjoyed my independence, and the thought of driving a car again (which didn't scare me at all – it seemed natural to get behind the wheel) made me realise that I would need to know where I was going. I would also need to know where my friends lived. I decided that I should go through my address book and the street directory. I would re-learn the addresses of my friends and family and use the street directory to find out how to get to them. I knew it would take time to do it, but I was going to do my best. My approach to everything was logical and practical and I was very aware when I stuffed up. I became hard on myself and expected to get better quickly.

I kept getting disorientated when walking around our house. When I went to our bedroom, I would walk up the hallway and turn right into the boys' room. I'd feel confused and wonder where our room had gone. Our room was at the end of the hallway, so why was I turning right instead of walking straight ahead? Also, I had a number constantly rattling around in my head – 634916. Why was I thinking of that number? It must have been important. I considered that it may have been a phone number. I instantly thought of adding the number two to the front of it because I recalled having to do this to our home's phone number. This made the number 2634916. Being practical, I thought that if it was a phone number then it might be in my address book.

I found the book and upon opening it I could hear my mum's voice in my head saying, 'If you have any problems, ring Mr and Mrs Powell.' Well, 2634916 was the phone number of the Powells, the lovely neighbours who had lived across the road from us in Brisbane when I was a child. I smiled at the memory and then the penny dropped. My bedroom in Brisbane had been down the hallway from our loungeroom, and on the right – the same location of the boys' room in my current home. I wasn't disorientated; I was living in the past.

Things started to make sense to me now. It sounded strange, but what if my 32-year-old body was living in Townsville yet part of my brain was living in the past, with me at 11 years of age in Brisbane? Like having puzzle pieces in front of me, I knew that I had found a starting place for putting myself back together. I would use my analytical

CHAPTER 9

skills and logic – honed by my years of work as an accountant – in my recovery. What I had to work with wasn't a previous tax return or a pile of bank statements, but it was real to me. I decided to identify each area to work on (whether it was an area of my body or an area of my brain). I knew that I could sort myself out. Finally, I'd be able to pick up all the pieces of my mind and put them back together.

Three weeks after returning home from hospital, I was starting to feel better about myself. I read the school newsletter and found a flyer within it. The flyer mentioned that a family was looking for volunteers to help their four-year-old daughter Monique, who had Down's syndrome and cerebral palsy. They needed three people to help 10 times a day with exercises called patterning and masking. These were to help Monique breathe on her own and to help her to crawl. Straight away, I wanted to help. I knew I could do something real and help others. Roland and Mum also thought it would be good for me and supported my decision. We contacted the family and organised for Roland to drop me off on his way to work and to pick me up at lunchtime. This was the start of a wonderful journey of making a difference in this young girl's life. It helped me in so many ways over the years, and I was able to see Monique grow up and achieve more than was ever expected.

It seemed that the only other times I left the house were to go to doctors' appointments or to have blood tests. On 16 September I had an appointment with my obstetrician, Dr S, for a follow-up on my caesarean. He was very happy to see me up and about, looking healthy. We laughed together when he checked my caesarean scar and said, 'Oh, it's even straight.' My reply was, 'So it should be!' We talked about everything that had happened. Just as Dr R had also said, Dr S told me that I had aged him 10 years when I became ill. Oh dear, I had caused the ageing of two doctors. I thanked him so much for everything and then his phone rang. A lady had gone into labour and he'd have to go. I overheard the name of the lady who was in labour – Susan. I said my friend's last name and Dr S nodded. Yes, it was my best friend from high school who was in labour. I told Dr S to go to look after my dear friend. Roland and I had to get home quickly to paint the cot (that was in our shed) for Susan's baby, because we had promised Susan that we would do that.

Dr S headed off to deliver my girlfriend's first baby. We had been best friends since we were 12 years of age and our birthdays were

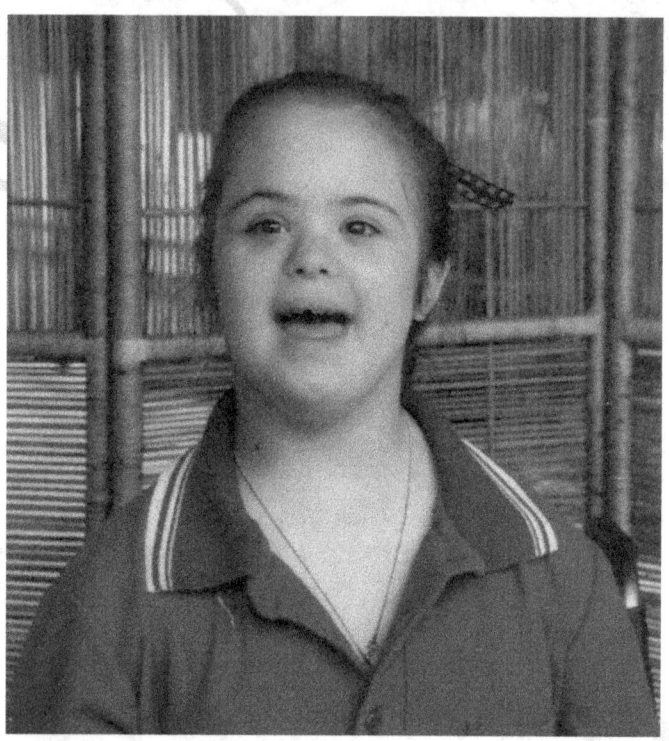
Monique (age 10), who taught me so much

CHAPTER 9

two days apart. Susan and I spent all day together at school and rang each other every night. We went almost everywhere together. It was at Susan's place that Roland saw me for the first time, and I was there for her before and after her first date with her now husband. We were married two weeks apart. There were so many memories of our time together that I would need to find and remember. I believe that friends are the family you choose. At this time in my life, I would discover how much I needed these friendships to help me find myself. They were part of the gold that was reconnecting the broken pieces of my life – they were crucial in helping me rebuild my life.

———————

Chapter 10

My mum had been so strong for us all and had done a wonderful job of taking care of us. However, the strain of the past six weeks had started to drain her. She had a life and a husband to return to. I wasn't well enough to take over without help, so my awesome sister Joanne made her way up to stay with us over the school holidays and ended up staying for three weeks. The boys were excited to have Aunty Joanne visit us, but were sad that Nanna was leaving.

Joanne could see that I was struggling to cope with day-to-day life but I was doing better than I had been – and I was more alert. It was so good to have her with me. A mum is great but a sister is awesome because we think in the same way and laugh at the same things, and we can tease each other and not get upset. It was also helpful to have a new set of eyes witnessing my progress. Within the first couple of days, Joanne picked up that I had no sense of smell. Nobody had even considered this.

I had gone to the fridge to get a glass of water. Joanne opened the fridge after me and said, 'Oh, what is off in the fridge?' I replied, 'I didn't smell anything when I got my water.' Joanne thought for a moment. She asked me to open the fridge and tell her what I smelled. I did this, but I didn't smell anything. I then stuck my head further in the fridge, acting silly – but I still didn't smell anything. Joanne picked up the bad onion that she said smelled revolting

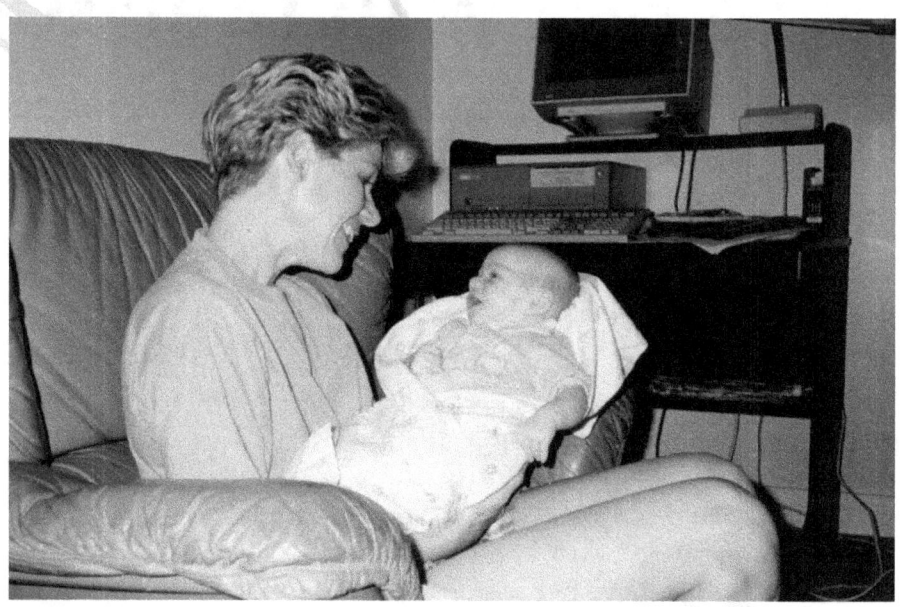
My sister Joanne and baby Jaiden in September 1994

CHAPTER 10

and held it to my nose. She asked me to smell it. Tears of realisation swelled in my eyes as she held the onion a millimetre from my nose and I couldn't smell anything. Joanne put down the onion and hugged me.

We started to check whether or not I could smell anything else. I could recognise the earthy scent of a potato but I couldn't smell my coffee. The air from my loved cup of coffee felt warm and thick but there was no smell emanating. Wow – how could nobody have checked this over the past six weeks? I was so upset at knowing that I had lost something else in my life. However, I now understood why Mum had complained about me not changing Jaiden's nappy when he had pooed. I hadn't been able to smell it, so I didn't know it had needed to be changed.

I had so many unanswered questions ... but, to be fair, I'd often forget what I wanted to ask my doctors. I wondered what else could be wrong with me and how I could fix it. So, I started writing lists that recorded my feelings, my problems and my goals, as well as questions for medical professionals such as my neurologist, GP, eye specialist and hearing specialist.

Since acquiring my injury, we had kept the general manager of my employer informed of my progress. Due to the severity of my illness and all of the unknowns, the company I worked for decided that it would be best to make a disability claim with my superannuation fund for income maintenance. This way, instead of me receiving 52 weeks of maternity leave, I would be paid for 104 weeks at 80% of my salary. At the end of this period, we would discuss my potential return to work. It was a relief to Roland and me to have the financial pressure lifted and to know that I had two years to fully concentrate on my recovery. I thanked my employer's management with my whole heart because they were looking after me.

Although I had Joanne with me, I was very aware that I needed to learn to do things myself. She wouldn't be with me forever. So, I started working on ways of remembering things. When walking the boys to school with Joanne, I started counting the number of steps we took and noting which way to turn. There was nothing wrong with my hearing so I tried to remember the sounds my footsteps made as we walked. Was I walking on grass, bitumen, gravel, concrete or pavers? The sounds and the ways my feet moved on the ground changed at different points along the journey. Sometimes I would close my eyes while I walked – if I could remember how my body felt at a certain point on the journey, I would be able to re-orient myself. There are so many ways to memorise things, and I wanted to use as many strategies as possible to ensure that I didn't get lost or panic. I kept practising. My goal was to walk the boys to school confidently by myself, and to walk back in the afternoon to pick them up – and not become disorientated. I wanted to be the mum the boys remembered from before my injury.

Aunty Joanne was a primary school teacher, and in the afternoons she helped the boys with their homework. Imagine having your own tutor living with you! The boys should have got full marks for their homework. I *struggled* to understand their homework, and this upset me because I knew that I should have known how to do it. To escape my feelings of inadequacy and frustration I listened to music. It helped to relax me, soothe my mind and make me feel safe, meaning that I could face the world. It also stimulated my brain and reminded me of what I used to be able to do before the injury.

As mentioned previously, I often sat and listened to Phil Collins' music. Music also helped my mind focus on one thing. At this time, I still wasn't able to read a book because my short-term memory issues meant I couldn't make sense of what I was reading. Watching television was also too confusing because of my memory issues, and facial-recognition problems added to the confusion. The movement on screen was also too much for me – my brain couldn't cope. So, whenever the TV was on, I just sat there in my own little world.

One evening a TV station advertised that it was going to televise a Phil Collins concert. Roland said, 'I should videotape it so that you can watch it again later.' I am so glad that he taped it. My eyes were glued to the television for the first time since my brain injury. When watching the concert, I just focused on Phil. I sang along with all of the songs and for the first time in two months I wasn't reminded of my brain injury. I was happy, alive, singing and enjoying the concert. I was living in the moment and not worrying about remembering or forgetting. I could just be me, and that made me so happy.

These feelings went deep into my subconscious and I remembered that they were 'normal' feelings. I had felt them before and acted like this before. I should be able to watch TV and focus on

CHAPTER 10

one person. I should be able to enjoy watching a movie and not be concentrating as hard as I was, or feeling confused. In my mind I had a list of the things I could do in the past, and I knew how difficult it was to experience those things now. I felt that I should be able to do those things. So, I wrote another list of goals and documented my frustrations.

I watched and re-watched the video of the Phil Collins concert. I would concentrate on areas of the screen that I wanted to watch, and this would stop me being distracted by everything else on the screen. I could watch Phil's back-up singers or band members and then look back at Phil. I used this video to train my brain to do what I wanted it to do. I then used these techniques to watch a movie. Wanting to keep things simple, I chose a black-and-white movie featuring a minimal number of people. Yes, it was an old western. It was so easy to recognise the bad guys and the good guys. With their distinctive outfits and hats and without the confusion of colour, it was easy for me to know who was whom.

After watching a few of these movies, I graduated to watching more-modern westerns that were in colour. This added another layer of distraction, but by then I was used to focusing on the characters so it became easier to follow the stories. Another movie I enjoyed was about King Henry the Eighth. I had no problems telling the characters apart because they were larger than life. They all had their own costumes (which didn't change much) and different actions and peculiarities. My facial recognition issues were still bad, so concentrating on behaviour patterns and costumes helped me to tell which character was which.

Without realising it, by studying films I was also helping in my day-to-day life. I was training my brain to concentrate on one thing at a time and to look at behaviours and other triggers to help my memory. But all of this concentrated effort was exhausting. At the end of the day, when it all became too much, I would curl up in Roland's arms. This was the only place where I felt totally safe and where I could just be me.

We had so much to contend with outside our bedroom walls. Our bedroom was my safe area – I didn't have to pretend to be a certain person (ie, a wife, mother, daughter, friend or patient) or re-member anything. Making love was so natural, with neither of us having to worry about my memory or my brain injury. We could just be 'us', as we were before my brain injury. It was a time to pretend that everything was normal and OK. It was also a time to remind us of how much we meant to each other and how much we wanted to stay together. A time to gather our strength to face the world together.

Chapter 11

About six weeks into my recovery I was able to prepare basic meals, but none were done from memory. I also didn't know how hot to have the stove or how long to cook things for. I didn't remember what I had put in the oven or how long food had been in the oven. To help me, I had a piece of paper near the oven and wrote on it what was cooking, when I put the dish in the oven and how long it was to cook for. I used recipe books that listed everything step by step. Before starting a recipe, I would put all of the ingredients on the bench. This was a feat in itself – I would read the ingredient list, turn to the pantry to get an item, and promptly forget what I was meant to be getting. This was so frustrating. I knew that I should remember the items. To help me remember, I would repeat the name of each item over and over until I had picked it up.

My pantry had always been very organised, with everything in its place, and this helped me after my brain injury. Even now I can close my eyes and imagine where everything is. Thyme? Spice rack, second shelf, on the left, two jars in. This system helps when my husband is looking for something in the pantry; I can just call out instructions for him to find it. Before I start cooking, I have to have the ingredients ready in the quantities needed, in the order of use. Then I start cooking and do one step at a time. It is easy for me to remember where I am up to if a recipe has steps, but I get lost if the recipe is just one long narrative.

At almost seven weeks of age, Jaiden rolled over from his tummy to his back for the first time and Aunty Joanne was there to see it happen. There was no stopping the little boy who had had a rough start to life. Every week I was reminded of how lucky we were when I went to help the family of four-year-old Monique, who couldn't crawl or even roll over.

It was soon time for Joanne to return home. She had enjoyed her stay with us and I thanked her for all her help. My grandma was going to come up but there would be a two-week gap before she arrived. This would be a good trial run for me. I could do it.

By now I was more confident with doing day-to-day things around the house. Mum had started the routine and we all knew our jobs. It was easy for me to keep this routine going. Also, Joanne had helped me set things up so that I could be a little more independent. Yes, I would forget what I had done and have to check and re-check things, but I had notes everywhere and our boys were very good at helping me. Plus, we had a great group of friends who would visit and help out, if needed.

Getting ready to take Joanne to the airport, I realised that I hadn't worn any perfume since coming home from hospital seven weeks before. So, I picked up a bottle and sprayed some on. Shrieks came from the loungeroom. As I turned around, my two boys came running through the door, squealing loudly. They jumped up and landed on our bed with their faces lit up. 'Oh, you smell like mummy!' they said together.

Tears rolled down my cheeks as I leaned down and cuddled them both. It was another magical moment when all of the problems that we'd faced melted away. My boys were mine again. For this moment, I was the mum from before my illness; I was the mummy they knew.

The next morning, I walked the boys to school by myself. I pushed Jaiden in his pram, remembering the numbers of steps and the direction to take. 'Off we go – take 16 steps and turn right, then take 124 steps and turn left, and then take 47 steps and cross the road.' I felt relief when I saw the school crossing and the lovely lollipop couple who had been so kind to me. I chatted with them as we crossed the road, and after a hug the boys ran off to their classrooms. I wasn't yet ready to venture to their classrooms alone, but I knew that I would get there.

I then just had to turn around and reverse the process to get home. Helping me to retrace my steps were the sounds my feet

> *For this moment, I was the mum from before my illness; I was the mummy they knew.*

made on the bitumen and the grass. I also counted my steps. Before I knew it, I looked up and saw my neighbour's fence. Yes! I'd made it home all by myself, pushing the pram. Such a lovely feeling of accomplishment. Getting to school in the afternoon would be easy, and the boys would help me to walk home. It was only the morning walk home that worried me because I became disorientated when I turned around.

Since I had come home from hospital, our fabulous friend Robert (whose dad John had worked with Roland – see chapter 5 for more about John and Robert) had kept popping in to say, 'Hi' and to see how we were going. When he heard that my sister was leaving and that my grandma would be arriving in two weeks, all he had to do was tell his mum, Viv. If you have Italian friends, you'll know that everyone becomes family. As soon as Viv found out that we would have two weeks without help in the house, she rang Roland. She told him that on his way home from work that afternoon he had to pop in to her house to pick up dinner. Wow! How grateful we were. Now began a ritual where Roland would pick up our dinner every afternoon on his way home and at the same time give back the dishes from the night before. John and Viv are a beautiful couple who know what it's like to be ill and to recover. They started visiting us more and being there for me. I had people I could talk to who understood something of what I felt.

Grandma arrived, and I smile now because my every memory of her from that time is a happy one. She had always brightened my life and everyone called her Grandma. Poppa had passed away three years earlier and that had been the hardest thing I had ever had to cope with. I was so heartbroken that I cried for days. I even froze and couldn't get on the plane to fly down to South Australia for his funeral. Grandma understood when we rang her. She told me that on the morning of his passing, Poppa had come to me to say goodbye and hugged me before he left Earth. He knew it would be hard for me.

How did Grandma know that I had woken up very early on the morning of Poppa's death, sitting upright in bed and feeling confused because I'd felt warmth – as though I'd been hugged? When I had laid down to go back to sleep, the phone had rung with the terrible news of Poppa's passing. Poppa had come and hugged me before he left. How loved I felt. This little lady, who only came up to

> *She was my angel on Earth
> and I loved her so much.*

my armpit in height and who knew me so well, was so connected to life. She was a calming influence. She was my angel on Earth and I loved her so much.

Now my 75-year-old grandma sat feeding her great-grandson and smiling down at him. With her there I felt that everything would be OK. When I was little, she had made every day special and magical. The boys loved spending time with their great-grandma and enjoyed having her come with us as we walked to and from school.

My grandma was very prim and proper, in that she didn't swear or raise her voice. However, she didn't have airs and graces about her and she could fit in anywhere. There also wasn't a nasty bone in her body. The only time I ever heard Grandma sound angry was when I was about five and Joanne about eight. Joanne and I had been dancing and singing in the hallway while Poppa was watching TV. He had asked us – a little too loudly – to be quiet. Grandma stood in the doorway of the loungeroom and coarsely said, 'Shut up, Max.' She then walked straight past us to her room and shut her door. Well, Joanne and I froze and the house went totally quiet. We both looked up in fear at the ceiling, expecting the world to end right there and then. I smile at this memory – we were in shock because our grandma never spoke like that!

So, you can imagine Grandma's response to the calendar that I had on the wall when she stayed with us. A fireman friend had given us a 'firemen's calendar'. Yes, the type with the almost nude men on it. I did need a calendar, so I had hung it on the wall. Every time I went to write on it, I found a blank sticky note on the picture. I would peel it off, wondering who put it there. These sticky notes kept appearing on the calendar. I asked my grandma if she knew anything about them. She gave me a coy smile and tilted her head (which I knew meant she had done something), and merely said, 'I dressed him.'

Oh, you have to laugh at that. Here was my beautiful grandma, not complaining out loud about the semi-nude fireman on the calendar. All she did was place sticky notes near the right parts to make sure he was dressed properly. How precious!

At this time I sat at the table trying to sort out photos, and realised again that my short-term memory was almost non-existent. I kept forgetting how I was organising the piles of photos. I also

CHAPTER 11

hated not remembering who had just walked out the door. So, to improve my memory, and with my grandma's help, I started playing the card game called Patience. My grandparents had always played this to keep their minds alert. Roland and I had often played double-handed Patience, even playing it on airplanes or in hospital when I was in labour with the older two boys. We thought it should help me.

I got out a pack of cards and Grandma reminded me how to play. 'Yes,' I thought, 'this will be easy.' No, it wasn't. I laid out the cards correctly but then I couldn't remember which card went where or which one I had moved. Grandma encouraged me and said I'd work it out. I decided to work on red and black, from ace to king. All I had to worry about was getting each colour and number right. I played all day, and I was constantly frustrated with my progress. I dealt the next game as soon as I finished the previous one. Grandma smiled as she watched me.

Days passed and Roland worried that I had become fixated on this game. Grandma assured him that I was OK and that I was doing what I needed to do. To help me remember all of the cards, I laid them out and became familiar with each suit and colour. I started to play a full game, with four suits. To make my brain work correctly, I decided I was just going to sit there and keep playing. I was so determined. Before long, I could see that the repetition and effort was working, and my memory was starting to improve. My grandma looked at me and smiled, saying that she was reminded of the little girl who put her hands on her hips and said, 'I'll do it myself.' Grandma had been such a blessing with her visit. She had to go home eventually, but with her arms around me, she reassured me that she would be back. I looked forward to that.

I became more able to do day-to-day things. I could do things like cook, clean and get myself ready as long as I made everything into a pattern (much as I had done for remembering the walk to the boys' school). I also used numbers to help me. For example, I would remember that I had three items to put in the linen cupboard. I had 12 items in the washing machine and I had three loads to wash. I had four plates, therefore I needed four knives and four forks.

I felt a strong need to learn more about what had happened to me, my illness and the brain. This was a time before the internet was widely used, so I asked Roland to take me to the library. I needed to do some research and discover how I could improve my short-term memory and take back control of my brain and my life.

———————

Chapter 12

To start my research journey, I contacted the three hospitals that Jaiden and I had been in and asked for copies of my hospital files. To access the files, I had to complete a form. When I explained that I only wanted the files to read so that I could find out what had happened to me (because I had no real memory of it), staff at all three hospitals were so helpful. They asked me to come in when I received the files, and they would go through them with me and explain anything that I wanted to know. I thought that would be really useful.

At my next visit to Dr R, I asked him to explain my brain injury, show me the areas that had been affected, and let me know what an 'average' or 'normal' brain was able to do. It was so hard for me to test and improve my brain when I didn't know what it was meant to be capable of. How does an athlete know how fast they are if they don't have a stopwatch or a competitor, or if they don't have access to information about the fastest time recorded for their event? I didn't have guidelines and I needed something to compare myself to.

Dr R showed me the latest MRI of my brain, taken when I was in hospital, and he shook his head slowly and sadly. I was confused by this. He confessed that he had forgotten how bad my brain damage was. I was taken aback by this and by the look on his face as he stared at the picture of my brain. I could see him trying to fathom what or how to say anything to me. However, I needed facts to work with and Dr R knew that I was determined to get better.

My questions, and the answers:

1. **How much of my brain is damaged?**
   Dr R drew lines along the scan and estimated that about one-eighth – or 12.5% – of my brain was damaged. (To imagine the scale of the damage, divide a circle into quarters and then into quarters again. One-eighth is a large area.)

2. **Which area of my brain is damaged?**
   It is mainly the right temporal lobe, which has many functions.

3. **What does this part of the brain do?**
   The right temporal lobe controls short-term memory, perception, concentration, mobility, understanding, communication and language.

Basically, with this damage I shouldn't have been able to do all of the things that I had been doing. I should have been paralysed on my left side, and unable to speak or put together sentences. I shouldn't have had any balance or spatial awareness. I shouldn't have been able to touch my nose when I closed my eyes. (Go on, try it!) There are many more symptoms for right temporal lobe damage, but there was no full list that they could give me. I had rewired my brain to be able to do all of these things myself.

Dr R shook his head and looked at me as he told me how well I had done. He said that there are two types of patients. One is the person who doesn't know that they have a problem – this makes it hard for their loved ones and carers. The other is the person who knows that they have a problem – this makes it hard for them, but good for their loved ones and carers. I was the patient who knew that there was a problem. Dr R said that it was going to be hard for me, and he knew that I was hard on myself. He sent me off to have an EEG so we could see my brain activity. He wanted to check that there hadn't been any silent seizures and that all of the pathways to my brain were working as they should.

I believe that being informed cures fear. The more information I could discover about my brain's condition, the better I would be able to understand it and therefore fix it. So, I headed off to the

CHAPTER 12

library to find out more. On the days when I wasn't helping to care for Monique, Roland would drop me off in the morning and pick me up at lunchtime. I love libraries and having their books around me. It is comforting to feel the energy and knowledge of those books. I researched my way around the library and read textbooks, which was an easier task than I thought it would be. I wrote down as much as I could, and I also borrowed as many books as possible. I needed to understand encephalitis and how the brain functioned.

Chapter 13

While I waited to receive the hospital reports that I had requested, I concentrated on putting my life back together. I had felt like a stepmum to my boys, and I wanted to reconnect with them. I was having trouble coping with their homework, so our awesome neighbours Bruce and Sharon helped out (they were the neighbours who had looked after the boys when I was taken to hospital on that awful night all those months ago) – every afternoon the boys went next door to do their homework. This was a lovely time for our neighbours, and I thank them so much for their help. I also remember the day I had to ask Bruce to help me get our son Kyle down from our roof. Kyle's older brother Tyrnan had coaxed him to climb up the greenhouse and on to our house's roof with him; however, Kyle was scared of heights and couldn't get back down. Roland was at work so I rang Bruce who came straight over to help.

Robert always popped over after work to watch a movie with us. His mum and dad (John and Viv) were wonderful because they would pick me up each week and take me shopping. They knew that I wanted to do the shopping by myself so they gave me space to do that, all while keeping an eye out for me (given that I could become very disorientated). I wanted to feel like the old me who could do the shopping by myself. It was good to have friends help with this aspect of life – they were able to take a step back and allow me to be more independent, whereas my family had wanted to do the shopping for me.

One day I wanted to buy some new stockings. Viv stayed home with Jaiden, and John took me to the shopping centre. He showed me where the underwear shop was and I walked to it on my own. I felt empowered. I had done it myself! I purchased the stockings and walked out of the shop. Shit! Which way should I go? I had become disorientated as soon as I had walked out the door. So, I stood there and looked left and right. As I looked to my right, I saw a smile that I recognised, and a hand wave. There was John, giving me the space I needed and the security of waiting for me where I would be able to see him. I smiled, feeling very relieved and a little more confident as I walked towards him.

Although I was researching solutions and having success with the rebuilding of my skills, I really wanted to work on accessing my treasure trove of precious memories. All of my memories were like the proverbial favourite china bowl that had been dropped and was now in a million pieces. I loved those memories and I needed someone to help me pick up the pieces and put them in order, reconnecting them with gold lacquer. My memories up to the age of about 11 seemed to be in order; it was the following 20 years of memories that were fragmented.

The best person to help me piece them all together was Craig. He had known me the longest and had been there for so many of my memories. So, I decided to ring him, and we started to reminisce about the old days. Have you done this with friends? You sit around for hours, chatting and reminiscing ... Hours went by, and memories were reconnected whenever one of us said, 'Remember the trip to Cairns ... ?', 'Remember when Tim ... ?', 'What about the time we went to ... ?' and 'Remember your 21st ... ?' All of these 'Remember when?'s put my memories back together. I was reconstructing the beautiful broken bowl that was my brain. Each memory was precious, and Craig helped me place each one in the right year with the right people. The photo album in my mind was being put together. It was well past midnight when we ended the call. Telstra should have awarded us for having the longest phone call in history, but we both smile at the memory of it.

Speaking of making memories ... John Denver was scheduled to come to Townsville in November of 1994, just a few months after I had experienced my injury! I really wanted to go to his concert, but who could I go with? I wanted to feel safe and also to sing loudly, out

CHAPTER 13

of key. Your guess is correct – I could go with Susan, my friend from high school. Roland drove us there, and at the concert Susan and I sang loudly to all of John's songs. Oh, what a wonderful time we had. Roland picked us up after the concert and we sang all the way to Susan's home. Roland didn't mind at all. This was another moment when I felt totally like 'me' again.

Christmas was coming up fast, and Roland entered our off-road racing car into the stadium race at our local showgrounds. Life was starting to get back to normal. We went to his work's Christmas party, and everyone there was so happy to see me. Because we were outdoors, the noise wasn't too upsetting for me. It was lovely to watch my boys receive gifts and to see Santa hold Jaiden in his arms. A little bit of normality, and a special family moment.

So many things were happening as Christmas came closer. One day I brushed my hair and stared down at the brush, which was full of my hair. All of the drugs I had been (and were still) taking were making my beautiful, long blonde hair fall out. Would I become bald? Would my hair stop falling out? I was so upset and worried.

I was walking around more by then, and I noticed that I seemed to walk into things (usually on my right side) and I wondered why. Noises were still too much for me, and certain noises hurt my head. What was happening to me? My left eye started to twitch and my left cheek spasmed when I cried. Sometimes I felt a pulse move through my body, a strange sensation that was similar to when your chest moves in and out during breathing. It was so weird. These things were frightening me. Was I getting better, or was I getting worse? My anxiety went through the roof. It was as though a door closed outside me and locked me in.

I became agoraphobic, with a massive fear of going outside. I couldn't have anyone come to visit because my anxiety levels became too high. I felt closed in when anyone was in our home, and I just wanted to run away. But where would I run? It was the worst feeling and I felt so panicked. Roland was supportive, and because it was the school holidays, the boys were with me at home. They were helpful, but they were also noisy and moved a lot, which affected my head. Robert and many other friends would ring to see how I was, but I just wanted to hide from the world. I was scared of something, but didn't understand what it could be. My world had closed in.

I absorbed myself into music again, hoping that it could pull me out of the bad feeling. I sat on the lounge and watched the much-loved Phil Collins concert. As my body relaxed into the music, I watched Phil walk out on stage in front of thousands of people. He was smiling and he didn't look scared. I turned my head and looked out of my window. There was nobody outside the front of my house. I looked back at the television and thought that if Phil could walk out in front of thousands of people he didn't know, then why couldn't I walk out my front door when there wasn't anyone there?

I'm a practical person, so this made sense to me. I stood up and walked to my front door. The door that had held me prisoner for weeks. I took a deep breath and opened it. There was the outside world, and nobody was out there. With my heart was pounding, I turned the handle on the security-screen door and paused. For anyone who has bungee-jumped, this is the moment where you hold your breath and, with all your courage, take that step off the edge. My step was only to go outside my front door, but it took as much effort and courage as a first-time bungee jumper. I stood outside my home, on our front verandah, and I took a few deep breaths to calm me. I had done it! Nothing bad had happened. Nobody had grabbed me and I wasn't hurt. I was outside and it felt good to be there.

This big step didn't solve my anxiety, but it did help me to start *coping* with anxiety. I wrote another list of questions and took them to a psychologist. He said that everything I was experiencing was normal. Generally speaking, it takes 18 to 24 months after an injury before you can confidently be recovered. He asked me to allow my mind and body time to mend. He asked me to try to stay positive and not to evaluate myself, and he added that there was very little I could do at that stage to improve my recovery rate other than taking good care of myself.

I don't know how you feel about what the psychologist said, but to me it felt as though he was trying to put a wall around me. I wanted to yell, 'Don't you tell me to sit here and wait! Don't tell me that there is nothing I can do!' After that, the first thing I did was to make an appointment with my family doctor (who had known me since I was 11). I asked him for a referral to an audiometrist to check my hearing. I also asked him for a referral to a urologist to help stop the constant bladder infections I was experiencing. I then went to the

CHAPTER 13

bookstore and purchased a couple of books on coping with anxiety. I wasn't going to let my recovery 'just happen'. I was going to start taking control of my health and recovery in a more proactive way.

———————

Chapter 14

The audiometrist checked my hearing and I passed all of his tests, so he could only diagnose that my hearing was overly sensitive. Well, that didn't help because I already knew this.

The earliest appointment I could get for the urologist wasn't for another six months. We were feeling a little down about this delay, but when Roland and I went to the boys' school for parent-teacher interviews we met another set of parents – Dave and Jacqueline – who would become very dear friends. We chatted for a while, and because we got on really well, we exchanged phone numbers so that we could catch up again one day.

We all need to feel that we are achieving our goals, and a goal of Roland's was to get back into off-road racing. Before my illness, Roland and our mates had converted our short-wheel-base LandCruiser into an off-road racing vehicle, complete with roll cages and a five-point harness. We had planned for me to be his navigator (just like in the old days) after our baby was born, and while my illness had put a stop to my part in racing, it didn't mean that it had to stop Roland. The Burdekin Off-Roaders Race was held and Roland entered with Chris as navigator. They won second place in the standard class (which was for vehicles that were still road registered and able to be used as standard cars). Our sponsors were happy with the second-place win and so were we. It broke my heart that we couldn't race together, but I didn't want to hold Roland back.

Life became busier and I was finding it hard to do more than one thing at a time. Often, I accidently cut myself in the kitchen as I

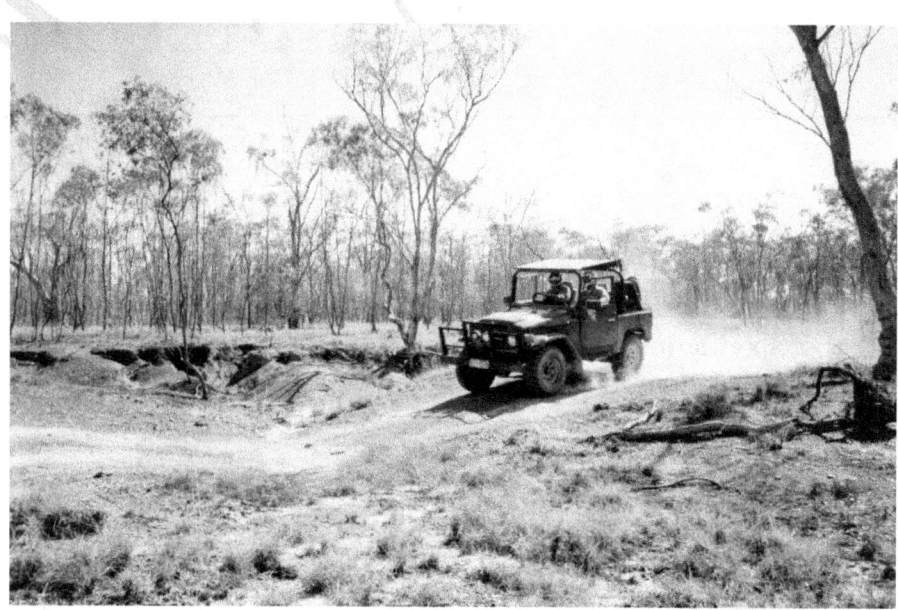
Roland doing what he loves – off-road car racing

CHAPTER 14

prepared dinner. Tyrnan was getting worried about me and before school he would ask me to be careful and to try to not cut myself. Oh, my precious son, so concerned for me. One afternoon he told me that he prayed at school that day that I wouldn't hurt myself. I was also walking into things, so I told myself that I had to work harder at becoming well and try to be a better mum. Roland would come home and often hear Phil Collins' music playing loudly as he approached the front door. When he walked in, he would stop to see what I was doing.

If I was sitting staring into space, he knew that my day had been really bad and that I was trying to change my mood with the music. It always worked and I would start to feel better and be able to cope – cope with the confusion, cope with all of the different noises, and cope with the flashbacks I'd been experiencing (these featured unpleasant feelings from the coma, and memories of being in hospital and struggling through my first weeks at home). Roland would come in and give me a hug and the time and space to feel better. If I was singing and smiling and maybe dancing, he knew that my day had been good and that he could come in and chat with me, just like in the old days. We laughingly called Phil Collins our marriage guidance councillor.

To our surprise, we heard that Phil Collins was coming to Australia in April 1995. Straight away, Roland bought us tickets to the concert in Brisbane. This would be the first time I had seen him live in concert and I was so looking forward to going. We would stay with my dad in Brisbane so that it wouldn't be too stressful for me. Oh, wow. This was awesome. It would be another dream come true, and having something to look forward to really lifted my spirits.

I had been working so hard to read and to remember what I had read. Each morning I would read the *Townsville Bulletin* and our other local newspapers. To help me, I started to cut out articles and piece of interest so that I could go back to them. On each item that I cut out, I would write the name of the newspaper and the date. My old auditing skills were coming to the fore again. The items were about people I knew; careers in accounting and management; taxation courses; fitness; children's activities; and health. I was trying to re-learn and absorb information to help me piece together my past and focus on what I wanted to do with my future.

———————— 66 ————————

It would be another dream come true, and having something to look forward to really lifted my spirits.

CHAPTER 14

One article in the *Advertiser*, from 1 March 1995, was titled 'Massage helps stressed bodies heal'. Another article, from *Independent News* on 26 July 1995, had the headline 'Australian Institute of Management has a big year planned' (in chapter 23 you'll find out how this impacted my life seven years later). 'Sleep well naturally' was an article dated 7 May 1995 from *The Sunday Mail*, and on 4 March 1995 there was an article from *The Courier Mail* – 'Brain injuries "hidden"' – that mentions a Maria Hennessy from Griffith University. This is the same Maria Hennessy I would be sitting in front of in three months' time at James Cook University (JCU) for my neuropsychological assessment. So many of the articles I cut from the papers were somehow part of my future.

Reading definitely became easier because of practising with the newspapers. The first book that I read after my injury was *River God* by Wilbur Smith. I had his complete collection and before my injury I had read them all. This book totally absorbed me. I found it so easy to delve into. Reading became just like it used to be. While reading the book, I could imagine the story as though it was a movie. I may have had to re-read some areas but I was getting my reading skills back and that made me very happy.

My medical reports arrived, and I made a time with each hospital to sit down with the nurses to go through them. I took a notepad and pen with me. Have you ever read hospital reports? What is it about doctors' handwriting? Nurses must go to the same school as doctors because it can be difficult to read and understand their writing, too. I rubbed my hands along the pages of my reports. These pages held the story of an important time in my life. They would give me insight into all of the days that I had missed. It was going to be hard to read – mentally and emotionally – but I was ready. I needed to know.

The staff at each hospital were so friendly and helpful. A few of the nurses that had looked after me were so happy to see me well. They showed me the rooms that I had been in and the equipment that had been used. Even though I didn't remember much about my time in hospital, being there made it real – it wasn't just a story that someone had made up. The nurses read my reports with me and explained the medical words and terms. I wrote notes so that I would remember this information later. The report shows the emotion of the doctors and the concern that they had. There is urgency, and so much care.

It was easier to read the reports' scary facts about my health emergency than it was to read what the medical professionals had said about Roland. There were entries saying, 'Husband concerned' (4 August 1994), 'HUSBAND DISTRAUGHT' – in capital letters in the middle of my report (6 August 1994) – and 'Husband present most of pm' (7 August 1994) … so many mentions of my husband. They were the ones that were so hard to read, because I realised how much my illness had affected him. To hear how much I had put him through … how could I ever make it up to him? Roland's answer was that I had made it up to him by coming back to him. I was alive and in his arms. That was all the payment he wanted.

Soon it was time to head off to Brisbane for the Phil Collins concert – oh, wow. I sat there mesmerised by the whole atmosphere and by the music. I didn't get up at the interval because I didn't want to miss anything. It was as though I was the only person in the room and I became totally absorbed by Phil's singing. If I close my eyes now, I can still see myself there, hear the music and feel the atmosphere. Phil Collins, thank you so much for coming to Australia at the best time for me. At the time when I needed you the most, you were here. What an experience.

The concert rejuvenated me, and made me even more determined to get 'me' back. After reading my medical reports, I decided to do more. I contacted our local university – James Cook University – and enquired about its psychology clinic. I also contacted Townsville hospital's mental health unit and made an appointment with its head of psychology, who had seen me while I was in the hospital. I also made a decision to get a new family doctor because I wanted a new set of eyes on my recovery.

I was taking charge.

Chapter 15

In April 1995 I visited the specialist clinic at Townsville's general hospital (now known as Townsville University Hospital) to see the head psychiatrist, Dr John Allan. It had been nine months since he had seen me in hospital. It was a lovely surprise for him when I walked through the door of his office. He was very happy with my progress and we talked about the issues I was having, including those with my short-term memory. I told him that my goal was to be 100% 'me' again and he smiled. He said that the key to my recovery would be to 'do one thing at a time'. Such simple advice, yet so powerful. I had the pleasure of meeting Dr Allan 20 years later at the official opening of a mental health building (I was a board member of Mental Illness Fellowship North Queensland, and the doctor was an invited guest), and I mentioned to him that I had remembered his wonderful advice.

The idea of doing one thing at a time might sound simple and sensible, but remember that I wanted a full recovery. I didn't want to take slow steps. Everything in my life had been turned upside down and I wanted to fix it. I was a mum, wife, friend, daughter, granddaughter, accountant and business associate, all rolled into one person. I wanted all of me back. I had worked in the corporate world. I had multi-tasked and prioritised to reach my targets. Why couldn't I multi-task and remember when I had stopped one task to start another? I often forgot where I was up to and had to start tasks again. I was very hard on myself and my doctors saw this and continually warned me against it. Even nowadays I have to remind myself to do one thing at a time – and to not be too hard on myself.

I trusted Dr Allan. He had been there for me since the beginning, so his next comment confused me. He said that he wouldn't be able to help me anymore. My heart sank. 'Why?' I asked, feeling rejected. He smiled and replied, 'I only look after those who have little hope. You, young lady, do not need me. You'll be OK. I will put you in the good hands of Dr Frank McDonald.' It took a while to take this in because it felt as though I was losing something and winning something at the same time. In that moment, Dr Allan boosted my self-confidence because I reasoned that if *he* believed in me, then so did I. I was going to be OK.

Once back at home, I never stopped trying. I pushed myself to return to the old me. I haven't yet told you about another issue I experienced from the time I came out of my coma – it was the fact that I found it hard to identify my emotions (they all felt similar), and this made me feel less like myself. Think about it from the experience of your own life – fear, anxiety, happiness, sadness and pain all change the way your body and mind feel. In the first few seconds of experiencing an emotion I found it hard to identify it. I was so sensitive that my feelings would become confused. Did I want to run, cry or smile? I didn't know. This upset me because I knew that I should know. Just as my doctors said, I was too hard on myself.

Friends often commented on how lucky I was to have Roland. This actually made me upset because, unintentionally, they were putting pressure on me to do better. Had they forgotten that I was lucky to be alive and that it wasn't my fault that I had fallen ill? They may have thought that I was doing well, but I interpreted their comments as meaning, 'You should be trying harder to get better so that things are easier for Roland.' So, I tried harder and did more.

Imagine having to re-learn each emotion. Smile, right now. (I mean it! Give me a smile!) Did you notice what happened? When you smile, your body relaxes, your heart rate slows and you start to feel good. Now think about a time when you hurt yourself. Express that memory in your body – your eyes may squint, your mouth may clench, your heart may pump faster and you may scrunch up your nose. Your shoulders may rise and your arms may hug your body. Try it. Now imagine that the smoke alarms in your home have gone off. Your heart rate may go up, and you may breathe in deeply while you

CHAPTER 15

decide whether or not to run and do something. Panic will most likely set in. Now imagine that you are a parent or grandparent and you see your child or grandchild get hurt. How would you react? It took time for me to analyse each situation and understand what I may be feeling.

A few months after my appointment with Dr Allan, my seven-year-old son ran to me one afternoon with a cut on his finger. He was crying, holding his finger in the air and yelling, 'Mummy!' Many of us have had this situation happen and instinctively know what to do, but I stared at my crying son's finger and I *didn't* know what to do. Questions were running around in my head: 'Do I hug the child? Do I hold his finger? What do I do with his finger?'

I became confused and went blank. Something in my brain told me that I should know what to do. My logical mind said, 'I am his mother and I should do something.' Yet my response was only, 'Go see your father.' This broke my heart because I knew that it was the wrong answer. I just couldn't cope with the situation. I felt stupid and frustrated, and upset because my brain injury had slapped me in the face again. Yes, I know that a brain injury can't slap you in the face. Yet, to me, anything that reminds me that I can't do something (that I know I could/should do) is like a slap in the face.

These events were separating me from my children. My sons remembered how great a mum I had been before the injury, so they grew distant from me. This upset me and made me feel more distant from the real world. I began to feel like a stepmum or, as I often said, 'an alien' – someone who had come to Earth and possessed a body. I didn't remember my children's favourite colours or what they were good at in school. I started to feel invisible. How, you ask? Well, as I've mentioned previously, my children did homework with our neighbours because I couldn't cope. If the boys hurt themselves, they called their dad. If they came to give me a hug, I recoiled and I didn't know why. Their noise upset my head, especially when they ran around inside the house. Basically, I was pushing them away, but I was doing so to help me cope.

When I was at home I seemed to function 'OK', and I pretended everything was going well. However, all of the noises I experienced (whether at home or out at places like shopping centres) were often too much and I felt as though I was going crazy. Also, my vision sometimes played up, but this started to upset me less over time –

> *I felt stupid and frustrated, and upset because my brain injury had slapped me in the face again.*

CHAPTER 15

this was because I knew that it was an issue with my brain making connections. I was still having trouble with writing and with starting one word yet finishing it with the end of the next word I wanted to write (eg, 'research information' could be written as 'researation'). This made for interesting reading.

Robert – the young guy who was like a brother to me – once asked if I could type up an assignment for him. With me being me, I straight away said that I would. I had been a good typist, so I thought nothing of it. Even so, I was surprised to discover that it was very easy for me to type. I found it to be much easier than writing. I wondered about this eye–hand coordination anomaly because I thought that writing should be similar to typing. I then realised that my fingers only had to walk the keyboard and not form each different letter, which is what you do when you write. It seemed that I was using a different part of my brain when I typed. I could type quickly and make very few mistakes. If I did make a mistake, my brain knew it and quickly corrected. Typing made me realise that if I could create a pattern for things then I could do them easily. I smile as I type this now because it was another win for my recovery.

In other ways at home, I started to feel more relaxed and in tune with my inner self. The family started to notice me say and do surprising things. For example, I'd be sitting with everyone in the loungeroom when I'd stand up suddenly and walk to the telephone. I'd place my hand over the phone, as if to pick it up, and then the phone would ring. I'd pick it up and chat to whomever was calling us. Everyone thought that this was spooky because I was doing it all the time. Sometimes I'd even say who was ringing us.

How did I know that the phone was going to ring? We wondered if the line of the telephone made a noise that only I heard. Perhaps, except I don't recall hearing a noise. How did I know who was going to ring? Maybe I was lucky in my predictions or I was good at guessing. These reasons, though logical, couldn't have told the whole story, because I was always correct. We have no idea why it happened.

Then there were the times when I would say things out of the blue and they would happen. For example, one day I called our sons inside and told them to clean their rooms because Robert would be arriving in an hour. They looked at me in an odd way because Robert had moved to Cairns, which is four hours away. None of us had spoken to Robert recently but I just knew that he was coming to visit. An hour later, he drove up our driveway to surprise us. He couldn't believe that we were ready for him. Such a lovely surprise for everyone. This is only one example of something that I predicted.

These predictions became like a game with our family and friends. They would ask me something to see if I could guess correctly. The question could be, 'How long before Roland arrives home?' I'd look at my watch and say, 'Seven minutes.' They would time it, and, sure enough, in seven minutes' time he had arrived home. I would also be quizzed about people outside of my direct family, and I would always get those predictions right, too. This was all fun, but I was curious about why this was happening and what my brain was doing.

I made an appointment at the James Cook University Psychology Clinic, which had recently opened. This is a training clinic for provisionally registered psychologists. Here was another uncanny moment, with me finding myself sitting in front of Maria Hennessy, the person I had discovered in the article that I had cut out of the newspaper months before. The article said Maria worked at Griffith University in Brisbane, which was 1371km from us. I hadn't known that she was now in Townsville. So many coincidences were happening. I became involved with places mentioned in the newspaper clippings that I had filed away (including ballroom dancing classes), or I met people featured in those articles.

At the JCU Psychology Clinic I outlined the strange experiences I had had as a result of my brain injury, and the staff were able to give me some answers. In the beginning, we worked on basic issues I was having in relation to behaviour, comprehension, memory, disorientation, hearing, concentration, distance measurement, and needing precise instructions and giving precise replies. These areas cover the basics of life and I had to piece them together one at a time. The good thing about attending a university clinic was that staff were able research my questions and come back with possible answers. I found this very helpful.

Here's an example of how my mind worked – if someone asks you if you have read the newspaper, do you say no because you haven't read every word in the paper? Or do you say yes because you looked through it? Because I had to listen carefully to what people said and wanted to answer correctly, this task was difficult. I still have this issue. Try listening to every word that people say and interpreting their words in a literal way – you'll be surprised at how often

CHAPTER 15

people don't mean exactly what they are saying (eg, 'See you later' doesn't necessarily mean that they will see you later!). For me, at the time, I was re-learning almost everything and wanted to get it 100% right. I wanted to be perfect but I became confused. A friend would say, 'Oh, it's a lovely sunny day,' but it was actually raining outside. Also, when asked what time it was, I would have to be precise – I'd check the clock and say that it was 3.27pm. However, all the asker probably wanted to know was that it was after 3pm or that it was mid-afternoon. See what I mean?

Another example is when you are asked to 'stand there'. I'd think, 'Which direction do I have to face?' 'Do I have to stand at attention or be relaxed?' 'What do I do with my hands?' 'How long do I need to stand here?' 'Do I need to do or say something?' Imagine this type of thought process happening in your everyday life and how stressful this would be.

———

Chapter 16

My attention to detail was helping me to cope but was also causing me issues. Getting up in the morning, I would have to do things in the same order and in the same way to know that I had done everything correctly. While protecting me, this safety zone was also the cause of my anxiety and restrictions. I couldn't function outside my own guidelines and they became too restrictive. For example, I could only be a passenger in a car that had my husband as the driver. If I went in a car with someone else, I felt anxious, even if I had driven with them before my brain injury. However, visits with Dr McDonald helped me because we spoke about stress management, personality types and anxiety.

I am logical and analytical, so after my injury it was easy for me to notice when I was exhibiting different personality types. When applying for jobs before my brain injury I had done personality tests such as the Myers-Briggs test, and re-doing such tests helped me to understand myself all over again. One test result said that I was a charming, warm and enthusiastic person (as well as being highly gifted). It said that I often generated new ideas, that I was able to influence people to take action, and that I liked to be organised and to plan ahead. It also said that I followed through on my commitments, and that I was able to handle complex situations and the juggling of data – all while exhibiting consummate people skills.

I decided that if my pre-injury answers to a personality test showed I had certain personality traits, I should be able to retrain my brain to reflect that personality, the personality that was innately me. To help with this, Dr McDonald and I talked about the use of positive words, with us changing my self-talk from things like 'I am a failure' to 'I am failing at this task.' I was told not to be so hard on myself. Dr McDonald wasn't the first to say this to me, and he wouldn't be the last. It was great that he understood how I felt.

When your world falls apart, it is often so hard to find people who understand you, without judgement. I was lucky that I had a great medical team, with a neurologist and psychologist who understood me. They saw past my injury and saw my strengths and determination. They did their best to help me with solutions. A lot of the time, I couldn't objectively identify the root of my problems, and this was compounded by the fact that I tried to cope with everything myself. I would notice that I had an issue but not realise that it was actually covering for another issue. For example, I knew that I didn't want to leave the house, but this problem only existed because I didn't want to get lost and I didn't want to ask for help.

I have always loved being the 'hostess' and having friends and family over for parties, so another way for me to cope and feel included was to have people at our home. I didn't know how to talk in a social setting. I didn't know what to say or how to say it, or when I should talk. I didn't know how loud my voice was because it always seemed loud to me – plus, what tone should I use? It was easier for me to be the hostess and to ask everyone if they would like a drink or something to eat and to serve them. This gave me a role to play, and I felt comfortable in that role.

I kept hearing from doctors, psychologists and my neurologist that I had done so well and achieved so much. However, instead of feeling good about this, I felt that there must be a sign over my head telling everyone that I had a brain injury and wasn't good at anything. I believed that people could see my faults. I worked extra hard to make sure that people saw me as being OK, or normal, or just like them.

We all need to feel included or useful. I felt this way when I went to help Monique (the little girl with Down's syndrome and cerebral palsy). It felt good to have a role, to feel useful and to help someone else. It also took the focus off of me. There was a group of us helping Monique, and after a while we realised that we needed more funds. So, we decided to start the 'Monique Robinson Trust Fund', which

CHAPTER 16

would allow us to raise money – and any donations would be tax deductible. The trust fund could help Monique to achieve her goals and help with her increasing medical expenses.

We had a great team of helpers, as well as three community-minded trustees. I put up my hand to be the trust fund's treasurer and to help with fundraising. We held cake stalls, sausage sizzles and cent sales. We spoke with local community organisations who helped with car modifications and equipment. Businesses donated money to help with the various operations that Monique needed. All of us were out there helping this young girl to have a good quality of life. We take life for granted but when you see others struggle it makes you realise what is really important and how lucky we are.

I performed well when helping others outside of the family, but playing the role of mum was hard. I mentioned earlier that I felt as though I wasn't coping as a mum. Well, even after exploring my brain function more deeply, I still found it hard to connect with my children. I pushed them away. I didn't know how to interact with them. I wished the world would stop and let me catch up, and then I could start up again. The only problem was, my children kept growing, changing and needing different things. I would learn how to cope at one level and before I knew it they would be at the next level. It was like trying to catch up to your children when you are all out walking – the moment you catch up to them, they race ahead and then you are behind again. This was a constant loop for me. My children wanted more from me than I knew how to give. I felt so distant from them and it was so upsetting. I didn't know how to fix it.

I mentioned previously that since leaving hospital I had suffered from continuous bladder infections and was constantly in pain. I'd go back time and again to our family doctor for more antibiotics. It felt like a never-ending cycle. I asked the doctor for a referral to a urologist, but he said that there would be a six- to 12-month wait, so he didn't give me a referral. A few days later, I was speaking with friends about this and they said that I should have been given a referral so that the process could begin. They suggested that I should find another doctor. So, I decided that, after having had the same doctor for around 20 years, it was time to change. I needed a new set of eyes on my problems. I started to look out for a new doctor.

Chapter 17

As luck would have it, I found a great doctor who was a mother and a wife as well as a doctor. I later found out that she could also sing. At my first visit she listened to my concerns and when I mentioned my hearing issues, she stopped me. She asked me lots of questions, and even asked which side of my head I protected. 'My left side,' I replied, and her next comment surprised me. She asked if I pushed away my children because their breathing was too loud for my ear. I stopped and thought about what happened at home. I answered, 'Yes, maybe I do.' The doctor explained that I had hyperacusis in my left ear, which meant that things sounded louder than they should and it was harder for me to block out certain noises (meaning that I heard everything).

Now I was beginning to understand what had tormented me for the past 11 months. I was hearing everything: the cars on the road 2km away; the boys clicking the buttons on their games in their bedrooms and whispering to each other; the breathing of everyone; and the sounds of doors opening and closing and the air being pushed by the doors. Earplugs were no use because I'd hear each heartbeat and the blood pulsing in my veins. I'd hear all of the noises in my body, including the gurgle of my stomach. Every noise was audible to me – even the noise of our dog running on grass. Receiving the diagnosis wasn't a solution, but I now had something that I could work on.

My new doctor explained so much to me in that first visit. She drew diagrams to explain things and she asked me a lot of questions so she that got the full picture. She even let me know why my hair had been falling out (it was due to medications and the stress on my body), and she reassured me that I wouldn't go bald. She also explained the rash on my hand and chest. I understood better all of the side effects of my medication. At the end, we made a follow-up appointment and the doctor gave me a hug, telling me that I was a remarkable young lady.

At the next appointment I asked about my constant bladder infections. After asking me a few questions, the doctor suggested that I see a specialist. She was concerned that the infections were related to me having had a catheter in place for a long period when I was in the coma in hospital. She made a call to the urologist and got the same response as my previous doctor about the long waiting time for an appointment. After hanging up she smiled at me and said, 'Don't worry. I'll give the urologist a call after work and we'll have a chat. I will let you know what he says.'

My doctor rang me the next day to let me know that she had spoken to the urologist. He had said that he would place me on priority and phone me as soon as they had an appointment. Six weeks later, I received a phone call to say I had an appointment on the Friday of that week (and had to have a blood test on the Wednesday). It would be on 4 August 1995, which was exactly one year since I'd gone into hospital with encephalitis. At the appointment, the urologist booked me in immediately for surgery on the Monday. He assured me that it would only be a day surgery and that all they were going to do was expand my bladder and rinse it out. He explained that bacteria was lying in the creases of my bladder, causing reoccurrence of infection. I was happy that something was being done.

I had no time to be scared because my mum had arrived the week before and we were getting ready to celebrate Jaiden's first birthday. There would be a party to celebrate one year of survival for me and one year of life for our son. I didn't have the time or the energy to tell anyone about my forthcoming surgery. We all enjoyed the weekend, with there being much laughter and many presents for Jaiden.

On the Monday – a year after getting encephalitis and nearly dying – I was back in hospital ... but it was only for a day and it was to fix something. It wasn't the anniversary present I had been expecting

CHAPTER 17

but it was appreciated. The staff at the hospital made me feel very comfortable and they assured me that I'd be fine. All I asked of the anaesthetist was to make sure that I didn't wake up during surgery (I think most of us ask this!) and he assured me that I wouldn't. So off to sleep I went ... My surgery was a success.

I don't do things by halves, and this month was no different. The day after surgery, I visited Dr R (the neurologist) for a check-up, and I thanked him for his referral to JCU for psychometric testing. On 10 August I went to JCU to start the process – the tests are done over a week to give you time to rest in between. The person testing me – Jo Wale, an awesome and respected psychologist – checked for general cognitive abilities such as understanding words and their meanings, basic maths skills, eye–hand coordination, complex planning and problem-solving, learning, memory (with verbal and visual information), facial recognition, and general knowledge.

I had a need to see what my brain was doing and to know how my brain function compared to everyone else's. I didn't want to rely on home tests or on people just telling me I was OK. The psychometric tests were full on and they stretched my brain. I bet they would stretch yours, too. Imagine being asked to remember numbers and repeat them back to a tester. First, you're asked to remember one number, and this then increases to remembering 10 different numbers in a row. You have to repeat them back to the tester straight away and then you have to wait a minute or two and repeat them. I got through that scenario, and then I had to repeat the numbered sequence backwards. Try looking at the following four numbers – 6 9 2 5 – and then closing your eyes and repeating them out loud. OK, now close your eyes and say the numbers in the reverse order. You had to pause a moment, didn't you? Now imagine having 10 numbers in a row said to you (not written down) and going through the same scenario. That's a little harder!

Another test involved a page of coloured or shaped items, with the tester tapping items in a certain order and me having to repeat the tapping in the same order. A related test involved the tester showing me a pattern, and taking it away. I then had to draw that pattern without being able to see it. That one could be fun – I could easily remember those patterns because they had a mathematical link (being shapes such as circles, squares and triangles). I was also shown individual pictures of people and then had to point them out

> *I had a need to see what my brain was doing and to know how my brain function compared to everyone else's.*

CHAPTER 17

in a line-up. Well, I could never be on a jury because I couldn't tell who was whom after such a quick look. This proved that my short-term memory and facial recognition abilities had been affected.

A certain test made me realise how my brain worked. The tester showed me a page that featured many individual pictures (just like in a children's book) such as a house, a tree, a door, a gate, a shovel, a hammer, a bucket, a pair of scissors, a car, a bike, a tractor, a bus, a book, a pencil, a table and a chair. You only have a short time to look at the page before it is covered up and you have to remember what was on the page.

For this test, my brain quickly worked out that there were 16 items on the page, featuring four categories comprising four related items. This made it easy for me to remember the four categories – house, tools, vehicles and school. I then only had to remember four items in each category. It was so helpful to realise the way in which my brain worked. For example, I would note that I had walked into a room with three items, or I needed to buy seven things at the shop, or I was going to two places on a particular day. I converted everything I did to numbers because it helped me to remember.

The testing's report noted that I needed time to devise a strategy for dealing with a task. The problem was that my brain was working at superior and high levels in many areas yet at average levels in others. Prior to my injury, my brain had been used to working at above-average levels, and it was having issues coping with the loss of function. The psychologist who performed the tests explained that if I was in highly structured situation where there was little distraction, my brain was able to compensate for my injuries. However, it still took a lot of effort to cope with everyday activities, even if I reduced distractions. She suggested that a structured program of writing and reading may be of benefit to me.

The psychologist said that, even with my injuries, my brain was functioning at a higher level than that of the average person. They wouldn't expect most people to achieve as much as I had achieved in the tests. I'm not sure if I experienced a feeling of relief at hearing this, or thought, 'Wow, I'm brainy!' It was great to see, on paper, how my brain worked. Finally, I understood more about myself, and this helped my confidence.

At this time, I also realised why I had become so reliant on routine. It helped me to get through my days and it was also why I found it easy to do anything structured and practical. The problem was, when a task included emotion, I went to pieces. Emotion added more variables – I wasn't sure how to act, what to say or what to do. Remember me mentioning that I couldn't function properly when my son cut his finger? This was because my emotion was part of the picture.

My best medicine was having my grandma visit. She made everything better, just by being there. Grandma didn't like flying so she would make the journey to us by popping on the train. She would tell me how lovely the journey was. Even thinking about my grandma makes me smile. We didn't have to do anything special, just be together and chat. We loved going for a coffee together. Our saying was, 'Shall we? Let's!', and we would giggle together just like the chipmunks used to in the cartoons we watched when I was little. Grandma would sprinkle her sugar on top of her cappuccino and we'd have a piece of cake. We acted like young girls, having fun and giggling. I loved those times.

However, my emotions went up and down as I tried to cope with all the changes my body and mind were going through. Each day felt new and I had to keep to my routine in order to deal with it all. A couple of times, I started to feel like the old me again. It was on those days that I wanted to stay awake all night so that I could enjoy feeling good and positive. When I went to bed, I didn't know if I would wake up feeling the same or having to rebuild myself. Yes, I usually had to rebuild myself each morning, and it was challenging. The couple we had met at the parent–teacher meeting months before (Dave and Jacqueline) rang and asked for help with their renovations. We popped over and realised just how much we had in common, and a great friendship began. They had heard about what had happened to me and Jacqui offered to pop over and treat me with reflexology.

Oh, how lucky I was to have reflexology every week. Massaging the feet helps to stimulate the brain. I mentioned to Jacqui that Pete had massaged my feet in hospital and she said that that was the best thing he could have done to help me recover. Jacqui would touch parts of my foot and ask me which areas of my body she was working on. Amazingly, I got it right each time. These treatments also helped me to relax, and they gave me the chance to talk to someone socially about my problems.

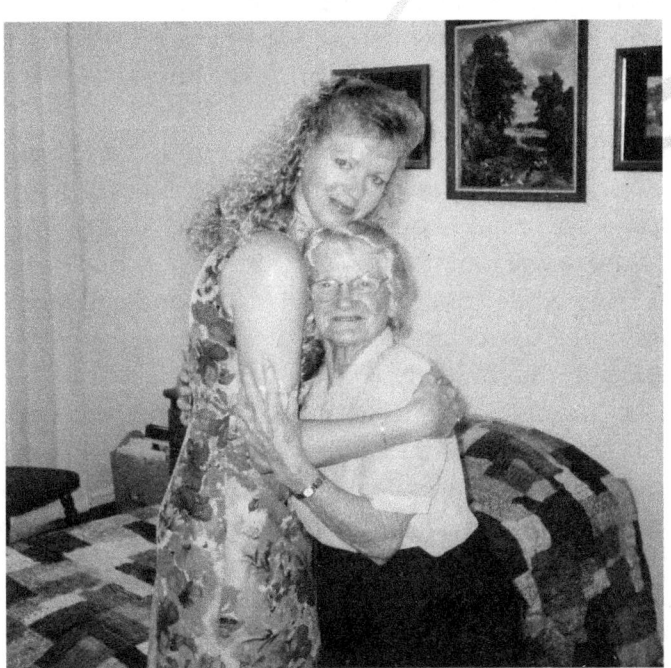

My grandma – the best medicine (and how I loved those cuddles)

Roland's work in the building industry had many after-hours social events and they always included the spouse. So, Roland and I went out regularly and I loved getting dressed up and going places together. Our neighbours loved babysitting our boys, which was fabulous. With so many doctor and specialist visits, I really enjoyed being with people at a social function and forgetting my problems. I only had a couple of issues when I was at a function – I became disorientated, so Roland would always keep an eye out for me (it's lucky that I'm tall), and I still had a big problem with facial recognition. To help with the latter issue, I kept close to Roland. He would say a person's name in the conversation so that I knew who we were talking to.

I found that I preferred the business meetings and functions where people wore name tags – it was so helpful to be able to glance down and read a person's name. One of my psychologists had given me some pointers on how to remember people's faces and names and while I did try these ideas, I found concentrating and remembering to be so laborious. It was also often noisy at events, which added to the difficulty.

I had no problems remembering my friends from before the injury. Around this time, a few girlfriends from my high school days organised for us to have a weekly craft morning. We'd go to each other's homes and sew. Oh, what lovely times. This was very helpful for the injured right side of my brain because it had to work with the left side. Also, craft and sewing were expressive and creative, which meant that what I made didn't have to be perfect. Being 'right' was an issue for me, because in my accounting world things were either right or wrong and I liked to have them be right. The girls showed me that you didn't have to be right and it didn't have to be perfect. It took a while for me to feel confident to make things, but it was reassuring and comforting being with friends who had known me for almost 20 years. They were so wonderful and they soon had me sewing and laughing along with them.

I did feel confident in some of my abilities. I was asked by a couple of friends if I could help them with their accounts. I said yes so confidently to their requests, which surprised me. It seemed that in my role as an accountant, I was more confident than in my role as a person. It amazed me that people who knew me before could see

CHAPTER 17

past my injury and ask me to help them with their financials. I loved this type of work and it was great to be able to start working again, even if it was only a couple of hours a week and it was in a relaxed manner. These friends had home offices, so this meant that I didn't feel the pressure of the corporate world and it was a way to test myself to see how I went.

I set up their accounting software in a way that made it easy for them and me to manage. This very structured approach made me feel like the old me. If you come from an accounting background, you might be interested to know that I went back to using journals and ledgers, as well as computer software. This meant that I had a great audit trail to work with. Depending on the clients' needs, I was working for them either weekly or monthly, so I had to make sure that I had everything working correctly and that I could remember what I had done. I wrote lists and ticked things off as I did them. This wasn't anything new, really, because I had always kept notes and made a routine at work. I was surprised at how easy it was to do my accounting work when compared to my many other roles (such as being a mum). It was as if it came naturally to me. My focus and concentration were excellent, as was my recall. I remembered accounting details and numbers and felt at peace; this was me.

Being the treasurer for the Monique Robinson Trust Fund also helped build my confidence and meant I was getting more experience with being in a social setting. Roland could see how happy I was at getting 'me' back but he was also concerned about my ability to go back to work full time. It had only been a year since my injury and the doctors were saying that full-time work would be too stressful for me – my brain had to work twice as hard to function and I became tired quickly. Dr R also wanted to give my brain time to heal, so I was to stay on my medication for another 12 months.

Our new GP also saw that Roland was showing signs that he wasn't coping as well as he thought he was. The pressures at work and at home were getting to him but he wouldn't admit it. After a few chats she convinced Roland to follow his heart and do what he wanted to do. He decided to start his own business. Previously, Roland had worked for himself for many years, and now was the time to do it again. He would set up the business and employ me as his accountant/office manager. Then, if the work was too much for me, he could employ someone to help. There would be no pressure on me, apart from the pressure I put on myself. We would make a good team.

———————

Chapter 18

We started 1996 with a fresh outlook on life, and I enjoyed setting up Roland's accounts and stationery and doing more things together. I still had my doctor visits and craft mornings and helped friends with their accounts. Family visited often and we went out with friends. I started to feel better about myself. We also went camping again. This was something that we always used to do but we hadn't done it since my injury. Easter was coming and Dave and Jacqui asked us to join them at Tully Heads with another couple. Yes, we'd love to!

How stressful this was for me. I had to re-learn how to prepare for camping. I took a blank piece of paper and wrote a complete list of everything we would need. I imagine it was like the list the astronauts wrote to go into space for the first time. Everything was on it, from knives and forks to sheets and airbeds. Once we were all packed, we headed off, towing our tinny (creek-fishing boat) because we needed its extra room to hold camping gear.

Dave and Jacqui had a family emergency, so they cancelled at the last minute. The other family had gone to the campsite earlier, and when we turned up only the older children from the family were there. Confused, we asked, 'Where's Mum and Dad?' Their reply was, 'They are up at the hospital because mum cut herself putting up the tent.' We were shocked at first, but this was just the first of many incidents over the weekend. Keys locked in the car. Melted Easter eggs. The king tide rising only metres from our tent.

I couldn't get to sleep because I was having panic attacks, so I asked God to make it so that I couldn't hear the waves. Be careful about what you ask for – within minutes of my prayers, it rained so hard that we couldn't hear the waves. Laugh if you'd like – our tent leaked and it rained so heavily that the men had to get up to remove the water pooling on our tents. It was the weekend from hell, yet we all had a great time. It was our first holiday with Ralph and Glenda and it wouldn't be our last. That weekend cemented our friendship and we've now been holidaying and caravanning together for over 25 years.

Over time, I started having more panic attacks, along with tunnel vision and ringing in my ears. My throat felt dry, and even when out shopping I felt claustrophobic and anxious. I even began to fear going to sleep. I became teary listening to songs because they reminded me of something. My doctor explained that grief is one of the stages of recovery. Nobody had explained that to me before. For the first year I had been too ill to understand what was going on. In the second year I was doing all that I could to recover and get 'me' back, yet I was so busy trying to live that I hadn't grieved for what had happened to me. Now I realised that some of my symptoms were related to feelings of loss and grief, and that these feelings were normal after a brain injury.

I had been thinking that I would be all better and back to 100% within two years. I became upset at seeing my original goal post move further away, knowing that it was doing so because of my bloody injury and my anxiety about it. How wrong was that?! On top of the ongoing effects of the injury, I was having to cope with depression, panic attacks and low self-esteem. It was like a kick in the bum. I was so distressed by this. Why now? Why me? These were questions that I hadn't asked before – I had been too sick. There were so many emotions going through my head.

Music helped me through this, as did the techniques my doctor had shown me and the information from books I read about anxiety. I often had Phil Collins' music playing in the background, and every now and then certain lyrics hit me. It was as though Phil was giving me messages such as 'hang in long enough', 'remember', 'one more night', 'can't turn back the years', 'take me home', 'against all odds', 'I'll help myself; it's up to me and no-one else.' Each song seemed to have a message for me and they gave me the strength to keep going.

CHAPTER 18

Because the second anniversary of my injury was coming up, in July 1996 Dr R ordered an MRI and a review. My doctor had sent him an update about what had been happening. Walking into Dr R's office was like seeing a friend. He was welcoming and understanding. I had had more blood tests and everything was going well. I was fine to come off my medication because the MRI showed no further damage and Dr R was happy with my progress. He checked the strength of my left side and he was happy with how it was going. It was a thorough visit and Dr R told me that I was good to go. He said that yes, I could drive again, and if I had any problems, I was to ring the office and come straight in. (I didn't know at the time, but his staff were told that if I called they were to put me through to him straight away.)

Woohoo! I was allowed to drive again! That put a smile on my face. Our family car had been cut up, painted red and turned into a fully registered four-wheel-drive off-road racing car. I could use it for my first drive, and I could feel safe driving it because it had a roll cage and a five-point harness and I had driven it before. For my first drive, I wanted to be alone so that I could concentrate. We would head to Pete's place, with me driving the racing car. Roland would wait a few minutes and then follow me in our sedan.

Upon getting into the car, I pushed my Phil Collins tape into the tape deck and started the engine. I asked Roland to stand at each corner of the car so that I could judge my distances. I then put on my seatbelt, turned up the music to loud and smiled before taking a deep breath and reversing out of our driveway. It was like being 'me' again. Phil's music was playing and I was driving my own car. I could hear my dad's voice in my head telling me how to drive, and I knew I'd be fine. I'd studied the street directory and had a piece of paper with a mud map on it, so I knew how to get to Pete's place. I had mitigated any issues and planned it right. Everything seemed natural to me. I listened to the engine, and changed gears when needed. Roland smiled and waved as I drove away. He gave me the space I needed to do it myself. He would meet me there.

Buckle up! The next part of my journey had just begun.

Chapter 19

It was an awesome feeling to be back in the driver's seat. I loved the feeling of freedom and of getting back my independence, which was so important to me. Being independent meant that I didn't have to rely on anyone to pick me up or drop me off. I felt just like I did when I received my licence at 17 years of age. Yes, I had a wonderful husband who would drive me anywhere, but I had always been an independent person who wanted to be able to do it herself. (I almost put my hands on my hips when I wrote that.) When driving, I could forget my issues and just be 'me'. My car would become one of my safe places, a place where I could get my head back together and lift my spirits.

Now that I could drive again, I could achieve more goals (including going back to study, and helping to drive when we went on holidays) and start to feel better about myself. I still had to plan my trips. I always had with me my trusty piece of paper, with pencil lines showing, for example, to take the second street on the left, the third street on the right, the next right and then find the seventh house on the left. They may have been stick drawings but I confidently followed them, without any problems. It would have been great to have had the easy GPS map systems that we now have on our phones and in our cars, but we didn't have them back then.

I would pop two-year-old Jaiden into the car and head off to the shops. Somehow, I would get the same carpark every time, and this made it easy to remember where my car was. Being a numbers person, I would convert its location to numbers – the fourth park in the third bay on the left. Just as I did with walking the boys to school, I would remember details of the walk from the car to the shops, including all the left and right turns, so that I could retrace my steps back to the car. Hard, you say? Not when you rely on this as your safety mechanism. I want you to stand up, close your eyes and take three steps forward. Go on; try it. How did your body react? Did you lean to the side? What noise did your feet make on the ground? Did you hear any other noises or feel any breeze on your skin? Which side was the noise on? These are the things that I now notice to help me with everything I do.

Our minds are fascinating. They can do and remember so much more than we realise. Each and every day I rely on my memory to be able to complete basic chores and the things that are expected of me. I compare myself to others all the time and am so hard on myself. Back then, I had to work out what was normal and then re-learn that normal behaviour. Once I even sat in a doctor's chair when he asked me to sit down. His reaction was funny – he became flustered and innocently said, 'That's my chair.' Obviously, nobody had done that to him before. As a child you are shown where to sit, and as an adult I had to re-learn this.

I'm not used to asking for help. I thought that if I did so, people would think I'm stupid. However, one day I saw a girlfriend of mine in the shopping centre carpark. She seemed confused so I asked her what the matter was. Her reply surprised me: 'I can't find my car!' Here was my very successful girlfriend, so confident and with no brain injury, unable to find her car. Lena had recently bought a new car and had run into the shops. She described her car to me and we laughed as we retraced her steps and found it. It was a reminder to me that it's OK to ask for help. I still need to remember this.

I so enjoyed being able to drive around, but I noticed that I was easily distracted by the noise of my sons arguing or talking loudly in the back seat. I had to concentrate so hard on the traffic, and on remembering where I was going, changing gears etc. There was so much to deal with, and being a practical person, I thought that it would be a good idea to buy an automatic car. This way I could eliminate gear changes – after all, I couldn't leave the boys behind to stop them distracting me! I enjoyed doing research for a new car, and off we went to shop for one. This was lots of fun and Roland made sure

CHAPTER 19

that all the salespeople spoke directly to me because it was to be my car. Every night for a few weeks we drove a different car home to help us make our decision.

The 1996 Mitsubishi Altera was our choice, and it had been nominated as the safest car of the year. It had the first road-sensitive gearbox, which meant that it worked out how you drove and responded accordingly. I had to try this – and, yes, it was really responsive to the way you drove. When going down a hill, I only had to touch the brake until the car was at the desired speed and it would stay at that speed. I ordered a metallic burgundy colour. I must say a big thank you to the guys at our local Mitsubishi dealership for making the purchasing journey so memorable. They would ring me and let me know where she was in production in Adelaide, when she was on her way to Townsville and when she arrived. In a way, the car's journey of being built and delivered reflected my journey of recovery. It represented the start of the next chapter of my life, a chapter in which I would become stronger and better. I loved every moment of driving that car.

The skills my dad had taught me when I learned to drive were so helpful when I took the Altera out on the road: know your vehicle, understand your limits, be seen, let people know what you are doing and, lastly, always make it home. Just as I had done with the off-road racing car, I asked Roland to stand at each corner of my car so that I could program the distance around it in my brain. When driving I had to re-learn the concepts of travelling at different speeds, calculating distance, braking, merging into traffic and parking. However, I had no trouble with merging on roundabouts because as a child I had practised synchronised motorbike riding (on our camping weekends) so that we could ride at events and showcase the newest motorbikes on the market. This skill proved helpful for driving a car on a roundabout.

I did get a bit anxious and confused at red lights. It seems that my racing background came to the fore here, because I expected everyone to take off as soon as the light turned green. However, everyone took off at different times. I would think, 'What is going on?! Get going! Didn't you think the light was going to change? How come you weren't ready for the light to go green?' I have to laugh because, for some reason, I didn't think about the green-light issue when my husband was driving. I had to learn patience when

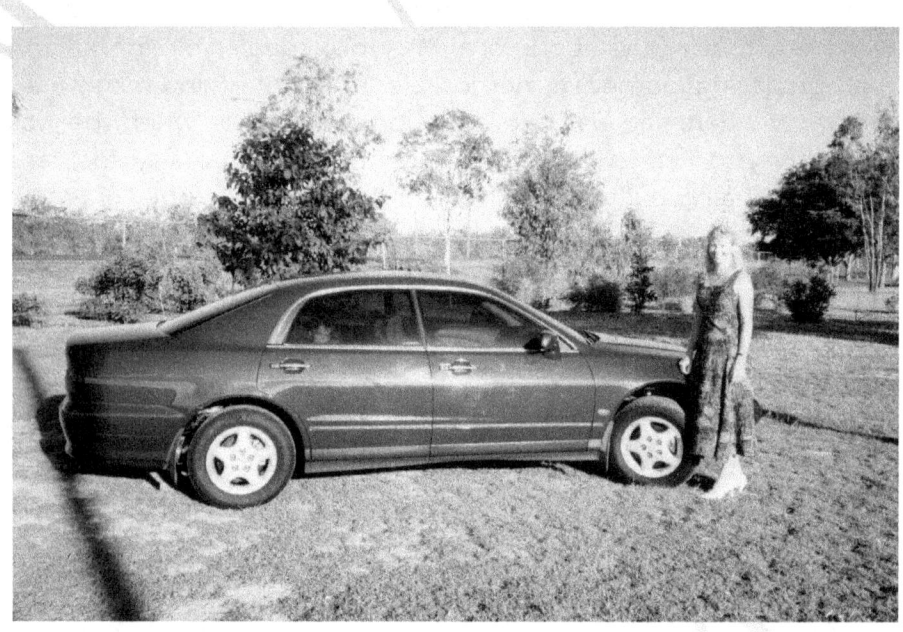

My Mitsubishi Magna Altera (named 'My Girl') in 1996 – another step towards independence

CHAPTER 19

I was driving, and calmly wait for everyone else to drive forward. I'm not impatient by nature but there was so much for me to re-learn. I imagine that it is similar to when you go to another country and have to drive on its roads with its rules, or have to drive on the opposite side of the road – it's a big learning curve.

I wanted to be responsible for my car, just like I used to be. So, I read the car's manual and in the back of my diary wrote down everything I needed to know and do. This included tyre pressure, tyre rotation, battery age and service timing. I also wanted to test the road-sensitive gearbox under various conditions – I took off fast and then slow, and I drove on different surfaces (even a dirt road). My car responded so well, but at the end of all of my testing I had to take her back to the dealer because the gearbox seemed to be acting up. The mechanic told me that I had confused the computer. He had never had that happen before. However, it wasn't a problem to fix it. He simply reset the computer and she then drove like a dream again.

How similar this was to what I was doing with my brain. I kept testing my brain and, in doing so, I confused it and pushed it to its limits. I did this so that I knew how it worked and how it performed in certain circumstances. The only difference between my new car and my brain was that my brain didn't have a reset function. Somehow, I'd have to find another way to do that.

To help with my anxiety while camping, we bought an old 18-foot Viscount caravan. Oh, to us she was a palace. Roland converted the front area into three bunk beds and we had a box air conditioner that slid in the front window. On our next camping trip, I didn't have to cope with a leaking mattress or a leaking tent. Everything had its place in the van, and this helped me cope because I could find everything. It was our little piece of heaven where I could relax and enjoy the holiday with everyone else. Before leaving for a camping trip, I still wrote up my six-page list of everything we needed to take with us and checked it off. After a while I became a bit savvy and placed my list in plastic sleeves, and used a chinagraph pencil to check off the items. This meant I could rub off the check marks and use the same list again next time. It was so much easier.

We thought only old people had caravans but we must have been onto something because all of our friends started to buy a caravan or camper trailer. We all were 'over' tenting, and our camping holidays became 'glamping holidays'. We booked them in for every long weekend, Easter and Christmas. Our camping group grew from two families to 17 families, at one time. Some of these friends I had known since I was a teenager. It was wonderful holidaying together and seeing our children grow up while visiting places all over Queensland. We still had those 'Remember when?' talks but now they were around a campfire. Card games were great, especially if you are like me and can count cards. I would try to predict what would be the next card or what would be the probability of the right one coming out. There was lots of laughter from everyone.

At that stage of my life we were creating special memories with our camping friends and our families – so many wonderful holidays and four-wheel-drive adventures – and I was ready for the next chapter.

Chapter 20

When looking at yourself and your life, there is a realisation that there are many facets to who you are. The businesswoman, the mum, the wife, the friend, the sister, the daughter, the granddaughter, the neighbour, the patient, the niece, the goddaughter ... and the list goes on. How do we act in each of these roles?

I had to re-learn my roles and I found that the confidence you have in different roles affects how you feel about yourself. For example, I felt confident as a goddaughter, and I knew that I was loved unconditionally. I remembered all of the wonderful holidays and times spent with my godparents, Aunty Daphne and Uncle Rob. For their 50th wedding anniversary, I made them an album of all of our photos together and photos of all the smiley gifts they had given me each year on the anniversary of my christening. For example, there was a keyring with a smiley face, a notebook with a smiley face, and a glass bowl with smiley faces all over it. I had kept them all. While I felt 100% confident in my roles as a goddaughter, granddaughter and accountant, I didn't feel that way about some of my other roles. Social confidence was an issue – I would sit back and not interact because everything happened too quickly for me to react.

Every morning, I had to reinvent myself. It took a lot of energy and emotion to get up and make a decision about what to wear. Unlike earlier in my healing journey, I now didn't have someone to help me make those decisions. I had to work it all out on my own. Which clothes went with this or that? Was it cold or warm that day?

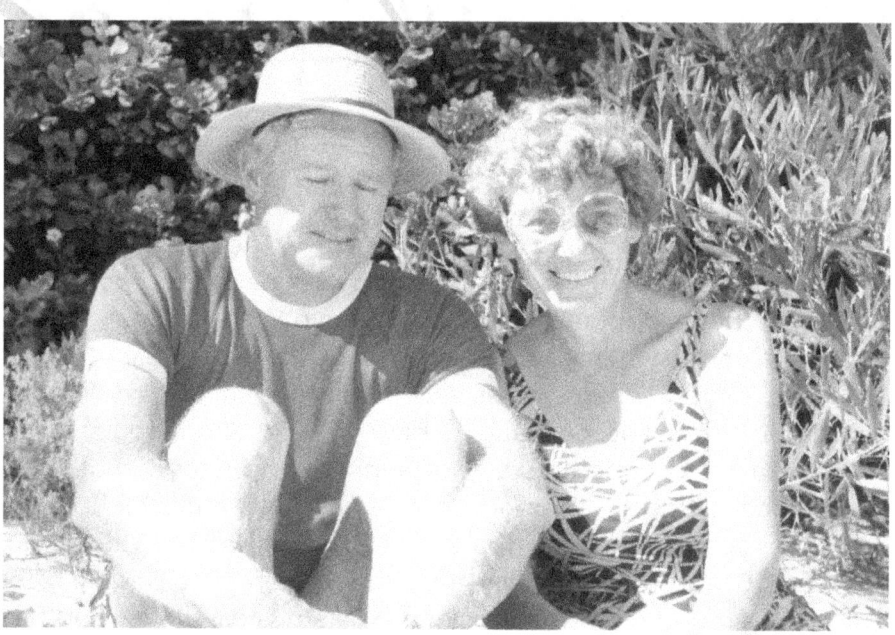
My special godparents Rob and Daphne in 1978, on one of our beachside holidays

CHAPTER 20

Did I need a jacket? Which underwear did I need? We all do this every morning, but when I first came home from hospital it was as though I was living in someone else's home. I didn't remember what clothes I had and which top went with certain skirts or shorts or slacks. This is all of the stuff that I had to re-learn. Life was like a journal and each page I turned to was blank, waiting to be written on.

I put together a step-by-step morning routine to help me get ready. By putting on certain clothes, it helped me to know who I would be that day, meaning that I would cope better with the day. If I put on my business clothes, I knew I would be in work mode. If I put on casual clothes, I knew it would be a day for more-casual activities. Different outfits allowed me to express different personalities. This system worked until my confidence grew to the point where I didn't need prompts to know how to act in certain roles. I also kept a bedside notebook in which I would write notes so that I remembered those items in the morning.

At the shops, I had to re-learn how to pick ripe fruit. Usually, you can tell a fruit's ripeness by its smell; however, because I couldn't smell the fruit, I had to work out another way. I did this by judging colour or texture, or by asking someone. It's often too hard to explain to someone why you want them to smell fruit for you, so I usually just guessed at ripeness levels. My tastebuds had to be reattuned to recognising flavour, texture and temperature, so I paid attention to noticing those whenever I ate.

Cooking was, and still is, also a challenge because of issues with smelling. I have to know what ingredients are being cooked and let my body respond to the smell. I often ask Roland to help with the identification of the smells, but I still do try it myself. I 'smell' the cooking food and wait until the name of a flavour comes into my head. I might think that the cooking needs a certain spice or sauce, and when I check with Roland he will often agree. I believe that I can smell but that I don't 'get' the smell. Complicated, I know. If I smell perfume, I wait for my body to respond. I have an 'mm' relaxed response or an 'I've-just-sniffed-a-chemical' response. I am very aware of these responses and also whether or not the air is thick or thin, or wet or dry. There is more for me to learn and I have a goal to be able to smell things properly again. I'd love to prove my medical team wrong because they have said that I won't get back my sense of smell. (At the time of writing, I have been noticing occasional hints of scent, so I'll keep working on it!)

Because I wanted to communicate better with people, I purchased the book called *The Definitive Book of Body Language* by Allan and Barbara Pease. This book is amazing and it helped me to understand people all over again. I started to practise some of the techniques, with me becoming more aware of how others expressed themselves and then responding in ways suggested by the book. It was fun! You can tell a lot about a person by the way they stand or sit, or hold their head or hands. As mothers we observe our children's body language closely to work out if they are telling us the truth or not. I still enjoy learning about body language.

Back then, I wore contact lenses. One day, while having my eyes checked, my optometrist said that I was wearing my contact lenses for too long each day and that I should wear my glasses more often. The contacts were the old type that you should only wear for up to about eight hours a day. However, I would forget to take them out. This optometrist's comment upset me because I was enjoying the freedom of wearing contact lenses. I remember waking up one morning and thinking that God had created a miracle because I could see clearly. I blinked and then realised that I had left in my contact lenses overnight. I told Roland that if they ever invented something that fixed your eyesight, I would use it.

I saw an article in the local paper about a LASIK surgery opening in Townsville, and excitedly I showed Roland. Oh, how I would love to not have to wear glasses or contact lenses. I rang up and made an appointment. The practice manager there, Wyndham, answered all of my questions at the initial interview and every question I asked at the next meeting. I passed all of the tests needed to be able to have the surgery. My dream to have surgery to correct my vision was going to be a reality on 12 March 1998. Wyndham met me when I arrived and the surgeon, Dr Lenton, talked me through the surgery so that I didn't feel scared. Wow – in under an hour it was all over. I was able to sit up and read the surgery's clock and marvel at being able to see everything clearly.

The next day I drove in to have my post-surgery check-up. Wyndham asked me if I had any problems, and he was shocked when my answer was yes. He looked so concerned, but I smiled and told him it was a problem that I wanted to stop to read all the signs

CHAPTER 20

as I drove to the appointment that morning. I knew that I could read them before, but now I could read them all without glasses. I told him that opening my eyes that morning had been like opening Christmas presents. I *loved* being able to see clearly. It was such an awesome feeling, and one that I appreciate every day. I was delighted when the clinic went on to write about me in their brochure!

———————

Chapter 21

Because we wanted to grow our business, Roland and I decided to become more involved in the business community. We were already members of the Housing Industry Association (HIA) and the Queensland Master Builders Association (QMBA; now known as Master Builders Queensland) and had attended many of their functions. Roland joined the HIA committee and we both joined Thuringowa Chamber of Commerce. (Thuringowa and Townsville were twin cities until 2008, when they amalgamated.) With me being me, I nominated for the Thuringowa Chamber of Commerce executive board and was accepted. I wanted to prove to myself that my brain injury wasn't going to stop me, and that I could be accepted by my peers. I didn't ask for any concessions and nobody knew about my injury.

I then put up my hand for the Chamber's event committee, and we went on to run so many wonderful events over the years. When our mayor at the time, Les Tyrell, said that he would like to hold local business awards, I put up my hand yet again and joined the small committee. I loved helping people and it felt good to be involved and achieving things. For this role, I was able to use the knowledge I had gained from attending many HIA and QMBA awards. We started planning the first Thuringowa Business Awards in 1998, and they were held in 1999. We had to choose categories, decide on a nomination process, create all of the forms, select a venue, organise the seating arrangements, plan the menu, find sponsors, work out sponsorship packages, produce judging questions, get people to be judges, organise media coverage, and so much more. These were awards for mum-and-dad businesses, which comprised most of the businesses in our city. We wanted to make sure that we held the event in Thuringowa, and that, as far as possible, all of our printed materials and trophies were made by local businesses.

The local WIN television station and *Townsville Bulletin* newspaper agreed to be our media sponsors and they went above and beyond to help us with the awards. Even on the night, the WIN TV crew were there to film the presentations, help compere the night and give a wonderful video presentation of all of the nominees and winners. The *Townsville Bulletin* photographer took photos of the winners to use in a featured section.

Over the following six years, my experience of being on the business award committee was wonderful. I spoke with all of the nominees and helped them through the process. I met with all of the judges and sponsors and worked with the media to get the best for our awards and our city. I wanted the event to run smoothly and be the best we could offer. Knowing that my memory could be an issue, I wrote down everything. I printed up the run sheets for the night, the list of all of the winners, the 'Winner is' cards and the category envelopes. I checked and double-checked to make sure that the right person or business was read out. I was standing nearby with my run sheet just in case something went wrong – but it didn't; everything ran smoothly.

At the final awards night before the amalgamation of the two cities, I was called up on stage to be thanked for all of my hard work and to be given a bottle of Champagne. They also made a special thank you to Roland for being so understanding about the hours that I had put into the awards. I had achieved so much and everyone in the room accepted me, for me. They had no idea when they first met me that only 10 years earlier my prognosis had been that if I woke from a coma, I probably would be paralysed down my left side and need to be looked after in a home, with 24/7 care. I had achieved so much but even now I forget this and keep trying to achieve more.

The day after the awards night, I received an email from WIN TV's commercial producer, and it summed up the night perfectly: 'Sandra, just wanted to say a big thank you, and a HUGE congratulations on Saturday night. All of the team have been involved in the event for

"

*The day after the awards night,
I received an email from WIN TV's
commercial producer ...*

the past few years, and we are all of the opinion that Saturday's was probably the best! Everyone we spoke to had a great time, and it looked fantastic! So, CONGRATULATIONS!!'

During those six years on the committee, I had also become a member of my school's Past Students' Association. It was comforting to go back to my school and its community because I felt a connection there. We were also building our new home and I was continuing to do bookkeeping for other people while running our business. I had a client who didn't want to change to a computer-based accounting system, and I understood this. I set up a computerised system that looked similar to manual ledgers, which is what she had been used to using. As a result, I had a very happy client who told me that she would enjoy not having to add up everything herself anymore. At the time, I thought that if I kept myself busy with work and community work, I wouldn't have time to worry about my problems.

However, as you know, problems don't go away and sometimes they become larger. I began having anxiety attacks when in traffic – I felt so closed in, which scared me. One day when driving with Roland, he decided to get our car washed. While going through the carwash I again felt claustrophobic, but I had an idea. Perhaps I could reduce those feelings by facing this situation again. So, alone, I took my car to the carwash. First, I bought an ice cream to give me something to focus on while in the carwash. The noise of the carwash and the claustrophobic feelings were there, but the distraction of eating the ice cream worked and helped to calm me. I continued to go through the carwash every week ... and it worked! Not only did I have a clean car, I also stopped having those anxiety attacks in traffic.

Chapter 22

I loved it when family came to visit, and it was extra special when my grandma visited. She would stay for four to six weeks at a time and we had such fun. Jaiden had started kindy in 1999 and his turn for 'show and tell' fell when his great-grandma was visiting. Jaiden decided to take his great-grandma to kindy as his show and tell exhibit. Oh, wow, it was a beautiful moment when Great-Grandma sat in front of the class. Jaiden introduced her and gave a short speech about how much fun she was. The children then got to ask her questions. 'How did you get to school?' 'What shoes did you wear?' One little girl asked her, 'Where did you get your handbag?' Afterwards, many children told us that they either didn't have any great-grandparents or grandparents or they didn't have any who lived locally. Great-Grandma was the best show and tell that day and it created a wonderful memory for us.

Around this time, I started experiencing odd sensations on the left side of my face. I noticed when the car's air-con blew on it, and touching my left cheek made the sensation worse. It got to the stage where I wanted to grab my left cheek and cut it off. No, I wouldn't actually have done that, but the feeling was so bad that I did consider it. At the time, the sensation also affected my concentration and my ability to think. This issue was very upsetting because I had been through so much. I didn't need any more problems. Then I started feeling a tingling down my left arm. I also noticed that my heart seemed to have a big thump every now and then.

I became really worried, so I made an appointment with my doctor who instantly referred me to my neurologist and a cardiologist for urgent appointments.

This led to tests, including an MRI, a CT scan, an electrocardiogram (ECG), an echocardiogram, a stress test and a 24-hour heart monitor. The cardiologist was very thorough and showed me that my heart was beating and working fine. One of the issues I had was caused by something I have probably had forever, but it was the first time I had heard of it. Apparently, I have an extra heartbeat. It can be a common occurrence but most people don't feel it. However, this alone wasn't causing the problem. Why did it feel as though someone was thumping my chest from the inside? He explained that having encephalitis had enlarged all of my organs and that this was probably why I could feel my heart thumping sometimes. This was another first. Nobody had told me that my organs were enlarged. This was a lot of take in. At least we knew that I had a good heart.

Next came the results from my neurologist, who was so worried about these symptoms. He reviewed my files, and because he knew my history, he was able to identify that the new symptoms were from a whiplash-type injury from a recent incident. There wasn't anything we could do to fix it. However, he suggested that we try medication to help me to stop feeling the pain from the nerve damage on the left side of my face. We tried a few medications but the only one that worked (which had needed government approval) gave me an allergic reaction that covered my body in lovely pink spots. I decided not to try any more drugs because they had various side effects. I had to learn to cope with the pain, along with everything else, and to remember not to touch the left side of my face because doing so prolonged the sensation. Some days it drove me crazy (it still does) and I also became depressed. I had enough to deal with already. Someone said that it was all in my mind and I cried. How could people be so cruel?

The anniversary of Roland asking me to be his girlfriend was coming up and, by chance, I saw an advert in the newspaper for beginner ballroom and Latin dance lessons. I showed Roland the ad, and gave him a 'Can we?' look. Roland told me that he had two left feet. I said that this was fine because I had two right ones. Smiling, he picked up the phone and enquired about the classes. The lady told him that the first class was scheduled for a certain date, and it

> *I saw an advert in the newspaper for beginner ballroom and Latin dance lessons.*

happened to be the night of our anniversary. I gave Roland a pleading 'Oh, please!' look. He asked the lady what time we should be there, and what we should wear. Fabulous! We headed off to our first class and we felt so welcome. Our teacher, Melissa, was great. She told us that if your foot gets stood on, then it shouldn't have been there. We had so much fun and met some lovely people. On the way home, I drew a diagram of the steps we had learned, and when we got home, we moved the furniture and tried to practise. Our boys thought we were crazy but we laughed a lot trying to remember our steps.

At home, I found it hard to do housework because I needed a routine and for areas to be organised. If the kitchen or loungeroom was a mess, it confused me and I had to clean up before I could sit down or use the kitchen. It was as though my brain was working out what everything was and trying to remember where the items went. It was overloaded. This happened so often that after a while I didn't have the energy to clean up. To cope, I went to my office or outside. I needed time to get myself settled. Some days it was as though I was a bottle of soft drink (soda) that had been shaken and was ready to explode. To fix this, all I needed to do was be still and wait until the bubbles dissipated. I expected too much of myself and couldn't face that I wasn't coping with basic day-to-day things. It came to the point where everyone in my little family pitched in to help me with the housework.

However, things were different in my role as an accountant. With that, I was in a controlled environment with organisation and quiet. Things stayed where I put them and I had a system in place. I loved my family, yet I felt as though I was pushing them away. I didn't understand why this was, at first. I later realised that it was due to the noise, the movement, the normal mess of a home – the cup on the bench, the clothes on the floor – and I wanted to be able to live with this. Nobody seemed to understand and I didn't know what to do about it.

The boys did help, including by doing their own washing. I would get confused about which clothes belonged to which son, and we had a separate basket and pegs for me so that I didn't have to find it when I did the washing. That basket stayed in the laundry. The boys had different coloured towels and sheets so that I knew whose were whose. These little solutions were so helpful for me. We all pitched

CHAPTER 22

in to make dinner and there was a list on the fridge for everyone to write down what they had used. This was a great help on shopping days because it meant that I knew what to buy – otherwise, I had to go through every drawer and cupboard and the fridge to work it out myself. The boys' cooking was so handy in later years when they were more independent and I'd left them at home – I'd be driving home and receive a message that said, 'Dinner is on.' They didn't go as far as keeping their rooms tidy, so we just kept their doors closed.

Our doctor gave us news that she was leaving town at the end of the year because her husband had received a promotion. We thanked her for all she had done for us. She told me that she would never forget my story and that she would tell others about it to inspire them to get better. I made her a patchwork wall hanging that said, 'Hugs, not Drugs,' and she hugged me goodbye and gave me a full copy of my medical file. I looked through the file and saw all of the drawings that she had created so that I could understand what had happened to me, and I saw all of her positive comments.

Now it would be time to find another good doctor, so I went about interviewing for a new GP. Life had made me realise that I needed to ask more questions and to find out the answers myself. The main question I asked when I rang and enquired at various surgeries was, 'If my child or one of us as parents gets sick, how do you cope with these last-minute bookings?' A couple of places said that they had a two-week wait for all appointments and some weren't taking new patients. When I sat in front of one of the doctors I'd rung, he asked me, 'What can I do for you?' My reply was, 'I'm interviewing for a new GP.' He looked up, moved his chair to a more friendly position and said, 'What would you like to know?' I had my file with me and we discussed what our family needed from a doctor and what help I would need with my brain injury, disorientation and facial recognition issues, and more. At the end of our discussion, he said, 'What do you think?' My reply was, 'I think you have five new patients.' My decision was reinforced when he opened the door of his office for me to leave and quietly said, 'Go left.' I smiled because I knew that he realised that I may be disorientated when leaving his office and not remember which was the way to the reception. We had found our new doctor.

Our home was always full of children and people. Yes, they were noisy, but it was lovely to watch them grow up, have a safe place to play, fix their cars and make me feel part of their lives. Some of our boys' friends even joined us on holidays. There were other times when I just wanted to have a simple life with Roland – just the two of us to go out together, and to sit and watch TV together. These were the times when I wasn't coping with the noise, or I had done too much in the day. Weather played a part, too, because my body doesn't regulate temperature very well and if I get too hot, I stop (like a car overheating). The feeling of not coping broke my heart because I had always wanted to be a mum and I loved my children.

───────────

Chapter 23

In 2001, I had more unanswered questions so I went back to the JCU Psychology Clinic to do another neuropsychology assessment. I wanted a manual for my brain, just like the one I had for my car. However, there isn't a manual, so I sought help. I was not coping with day-to-day life. The problem was that I seemed fine to everyone else, but I knew that I wasn't. I should have remembered lots of things that I didn't remember, and although I had been able to multi-task previously, I now couldn't. I was having trouble doing small tasks, and even having a shower could be stressful because I would forget if I had washed my face, or I would shampoo my hair three times because I had lost count. Nobody could see this, but I had high expectations and I felt bad about myself. I asked myself, 'If I act like this now, how will I be when I'm old?' This question frightened me.

This time my report included graphs. The vertical axis featured measurements of low-average, average, high-average and superior. The horizontal axis represented brain function. This graphical representation was what I needed to understand 'me'. The tests showed that I had superior perceptual organisation and processing speed but average verbal comprehension and high-average working memory. So, in those four areas, I was working on three different platforms or speeds. Imagine you are conducting an orchestra. The drummer and guitarist are playing at different speeds. The organist is playing a different song, while the singer is off-key and someone is playing a tambourine. This was how my brain was functioning. It knew that each part should be playing on the same level, at the same speed and in sync with the other parts, and it wasn't. I had to find ways of helping my brain to cope with this difference. As a start, one easy way was to give my brain time to find information, understand it, formulate a reply and take action on it. The biggest problem was getting me to slow down.

What would help me to structure my sentences and use the correct words and tone when speaking? I read about a speechcraft course being run by Townsville Toastmasters, and decided to enrol. The people there helped you to write concise speeches and talk in a safe environment – they all wanted to help you. This gave me more confidence when speaking to others, especially when talking about myself and my brain injury. Little did I know that this course would become invaluable to me in the next couple of years.

In 2002, I received a call from staff at the Australian Institute of Management (AIM), asking if I would like to join the local executive committee and help with their Management Excellence Awards (MEA). They had seen my work with the Thuringowa Business Awards. Oh, wow! Of course, I said yes, because it would be such a privilege. I was accepted as an associate fellow and once I was a member they asked if I would like to be part of the organisation's North Queensland Women in Management group. I joined that group, too, and it was wonderful to be around a great group of women. I later took on the role of the president of that group in 2004 and 2005.

That same year (2002), I accepted the nomination of president for The Cathedral School Past Students' Association (PSA). Now I *really* needed to be able to speak in front of hundreds of people. My heart might have been pounding and my knees shaking, but I loved that awesome, euphoric feeling you experience when you have finished giving a speech. I felt like pumping the air and yelling, 'Woohoo! I did it!' No, I didn't actually do this; I just gracefully left the stage to sit down. At home, I told my children that the PSA was the Parents' Snooping Association, which is why I always knew what they were up to at school. I'm not sure if they believed me.

Our oldest son Tyrnan graduated grade 12 that year, and it was my privilege to be a speaker at his formal, congratulating the graduating class. I had signed all of their graduation certificates and

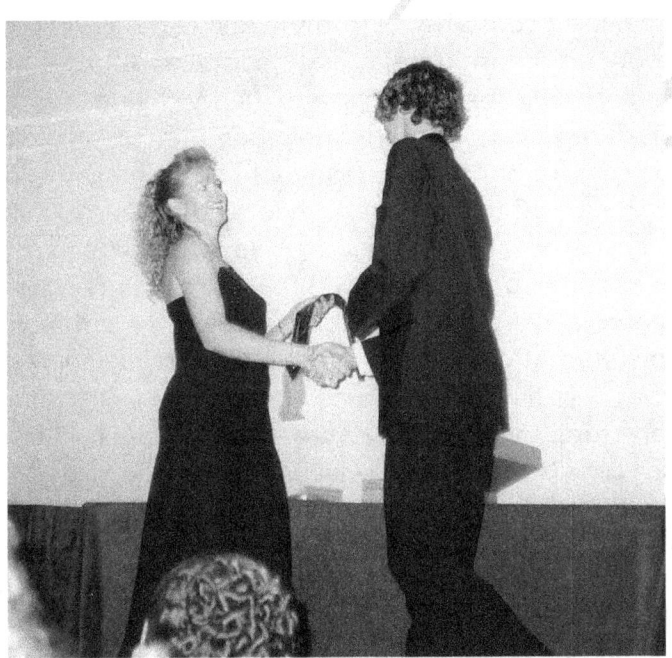

What an honour – congratulating my son Tyrnan on becoming a Past Student of Cathedral School

they came up on stage one at a time for me to shake their hand and welcome them as past students. It was a real privilege to hug my son on stage and congratulate him and all of his friends, who were like family to us. Being a VIP at this function also meant that my ticket as a parent could be given to my mum, Tyrnan's nanna. She was over the moon to be at her eldest grandson's formal. We giggle now at the photo of the class of 2002, because right at the top of the stairs is a little lady – Nanna. A fabulous unintentional photobomb.

I surrounded myself with good mentors and pushed myself to be the best person I could be. With my bookkeeping work for clients, and my work on committees, it had been a great experience to be alongside so many inspirational and hardworking people. In my home office there were different briefcases lined up (each a different colour, for easy identification), ready for me to grab the one that I needed and race off to a meeting. I had learned so much about our community and how to function as a person. I had been accepted in the business community and felt right at home in the boardroom. In these situations, everyone had a role to play; it was organised, structured and systematic. My organisational skills really helped me, and I knew what I needed to do and how to do it.

At work functions, people wore name tags, and that meant that I wasn't inconvenienced by facial recognition issues. I was also involved in the format of the evening, felt comfortable in the rooms because the events were often in familiar rooms, and knew the seating arrangement and format of the evening. Non-work functions were different, though, as there were no rules and I could become overwhelmed. In those instances, I checked out the room, noting where the toilets, bar, tables and exits were. I familiarised myself with where we were sitting so that I didn't become lost. It was OK if Roland was with me, but if I was alone, I didn't feel as confident. It became easier, over time. I pushed myself (and still do) so that I could feel more confident in all settings and be able to go to functions alone – I didn't necessarily want to go on my own, but it was good to know that I could.

Being at work (which was task-oriented) was so different to being at home. To make it easier, I tried to keep to a routine. This helped me to remember what I needed to do. I still found it hard to cook without using a recipe, because I didn't remember recipes. My memory issues made everything complicated and time-consuming,

CHAPTER 23

and reinforced that I had a brain injury. We even moved the furniture around so that my left side wasn't facing noisy areas. This helped my head. Everyone saw me as OK, but I imagined that they wouldn't last a day in my shoes. When things got too much for me, I still found that the best way to cope was by listening to Phil Collins' music. Sometimes I would tell Roland that I needed to go for a drive with Phil. Roland knew this meant that I wasn't coping and that I needed to go for a drive either along the Strand on Townsville's foreshore, or up to Hervey Range, with Phil's music playing loudly. This was like therapy for me because it soothed my mind and seemed to re-set my mood. (Music therapy is now used for many types of illnesses.)

My safe place was standing beside Keelbottom Creek on top of Hervey Range. As a kid I went there with my parents, as a teenager I went there with my friends, as a woman I went there with my husband, and I could also go there to cry because nobody heard me. Do you have a place to which you like to go? Maybe you like to go to the beach and watch the waves crashing onto the shore, walking along the sand with bare feet, and kicking it as you go along? I enjoyed that, too, but Hervey Range was a place that healed me and made me remember the good times. At home, I sometimes held the rock that I picked up from Keelbottom Creek on 2 September 1991, the day my grandfather passed away and I felt that my whole world had been destroyed. When I held the rock, I felt my strength return. Rocks represent strength, durability and reliability so, when I needed to, I held that rock to remind me of those qualities.

People judged me without understanding me. I had hired a personal trainer for 12 weeks of sessions at a gym, and people asked me why I needed one. They didn't ask whether everything was OK or what were my goals at the gym. If you had wanted to know, I would have told you that I hired the trainer because I became disorientated at the gym, and didn't know or remember how to work all of the equipment. If someone was using the equipment that I needed, I found it hard to change my routine and remember where I was up to. I had spatial recognition and balance issues so I needed help. If I went for a walk, I preferred to go with a girlfriend or sometimes with an occupational therapist because I could easily become disorientated. This upset me because I knew that I should be able to go to the gym or for a walk by myself.

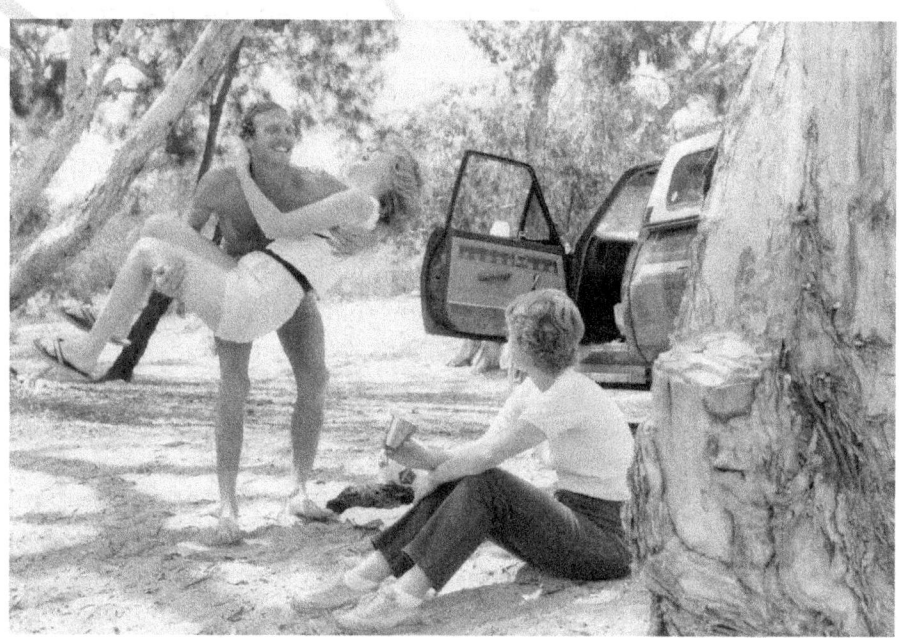

Roland and I at Keelbottom Creek way back in 1984 (no, he didn't drop me in the water), with Mum watching on

CHAPTER 23

I went back to playing golf, which I had played as a teenager. I started with a weekly ladies' group and when that disbanded I paired off with a lady from the group so that we could continue playing. I needed someone to come with me so that I didn't become disorientated on the golf course. No, I didn't tell any of my golfing friends about my brain injury because I didn't know how to ask for help, what to say or how to say it. I also didn't want people to know that I had an injury, and I was doing my best to try to forget it myself! I was becoming a great actress, able to convince everyone that I was OK ... everyone but myself, of course.

———————

Chapter 24

In 2003 I took another course in public speaking to give me a better understanding of how to put together speeches and talk without notes, and to give me memory tips. A couple of months later, I received a phone call asking me if I would be prepared to stand as an independent member for the state seat of Mundingburra here in Townsville. I said yes without really knowing what the role entailed. I had always wanted to do something for our community, and I would do my best as a member of parliament. On 9 August 2003, I met Bob Katter, the federal member for the electorate of Kennedy. Bob was an independent (until he started Katter's Australian Party later), and he wanted to discuss the forthcoming state election. He had been the sitting member since 1993 and wanted to share his knowledge and help others get into politics.

The next seven months were full on. I was nominated on 11 August, and the features manager at the *Townsville Bulletin* (with whom I had worked for the Thuringowa Business Awards) offered his knowledge by being my campaign manager. A fellow member of the AIM offered his help with my speeches and my promotional material. Without having to ask, people were offering to help me and I felt so privileged. We had many meetings with Bob Katter – he had a small group of independents whom he would help to stand for each state seat. We needed to write our policies, set up our campaign and be a team. We were all self-funded so funds were very limited. This was the start of Katter's Australian Party and it was a wonderful experience to walk the campaign with Bob.

He taught me how important your clothing is, because you need to make sure people feel comfortable talking with you. For example, you don't want a man's wife thinking, by your clothing choices, that you are chatting up her husband. You want people to take you seriously and you don't want them to feel that they can't approach you. My blue 'lady next door' dress worked well, and when I wore it, everyone I spoke to seemed relaxed and chatty. However, if I wore my business suit, they all looked at me and kept walking. Perhaps they thought that I was going to sell them something? Also, I was able to find out so much about what was going on in our community by chatting to people in shop queues. I was asked my opinions on abortion, gay marriage, motorbikes and bikies ... so many topics that people felt passionate about. This also helped me to see where I stood in regard to these topics. I was reading a lot and learning very quickly.

I also learned about ways in which to stand and sit so that you are better noticed by people – more body-language learning. Bob seemed to know and remember everyone's name, which surprised me. What surprised both of us was how many people I knew. Yes, I had facial recognition problems, but when Bob called out to someone and they started chatting, I realised that I might know their children. I would say, 'Oh, do you have a son called ...?' ' ... or a daughter ...?' Bob and I were from different generations and we had to laugh about that.

On one occasion I had to phone Bob while he was in Canberra. Bob had given us his direct line in case we needed him, and on this particular matter we did. I had watched a few old English movies, and the man who answered Bob's phone sounded like one of those movies' black-suited butlers. 'Bob Katter's office. How can I be of assistance to you?' I heard a very prim and proper voice say. I asked if I could speak to Bob and was told that he was out of the office. I was asked whether or not I would like to leave a message. I imagined this man having a serious look on his face. My reply was, 'Yes, please. Could you tell Bob that Sandy in Townsville rang.' I then had to smile as the gentleman on the other end of the phone asked, 'Is that all, then?', English accent and all. I could almost see the curious look on his face, and his tilted head. 'Yes,' was my reply. Bob did ring me back.

Chapter 25

The son of a friend of ours was very ill so they arranged a fund-raising ball to help with his medical expenses. It was held in the hall of a local school, so we all dressed up and put on our best faces. As it happens, it had rained that day, so there was a lot of water in the carpark. A group of us walking in from the carpark at the same time stopped as we reached the large expanse of not-quite-ankle-deep water. Nobody moved, and I looked up and down the line of people. Sometimes we need to be reminded to have fun, so I said to everyone, 'Hey, we are going to get wet anyway, so how about we enjoy it?' I could see smiles appearing on the faces around me and, as if on cue, we all stepped into the water with a splash and started to laugh. I still smile at this memory.

At the ball I sat next to a lady who became a dear friend. We hit it off straight away and she asked me if I would like to join her and another friend for an all-girls fishing team at the upcoming billfish tournament. I had seen the tournament's boats years before and had wanted to go on one. Roland encouraged me to push my limits and go. You can imagine how daunting it would be to have 12 hours on a boat, unable to see land in any direction. Would I become claustrophobic, or embarrass myself by having a panic attack? However, I said yes to going, and it was an amazing experience. We had a fabulous time on this catch-and-release tournament. Our team won the 'best dressed' award and I won the 'heaviest other fish' (other than billfish or sailfish) award on one of the days. I did push my limits but I had a very supportive team who accepted me for being me and doing my best.

Our sons played football and soccer and loved their sport. Roland and I both took them to practice, but for their games on weekends, Roland was often working so I had to take them alone. In the beginning the boys walked me to their field but as they grew older, they ran ahead of me. I became lost and couldn't remember which field they were on, and I was too self-conscious to ask for help. Instead of being honest with the boys and telling them what was happening, I tried to hide it. I started to drop them off from the car, saying that I had to go somewhere and that I would pick them up after the game. I would watch them walk away and when I knew they couldn't see me, I would move to another park within the carpark. Then, I would sit there trying not to cry. I didn't want my eyes to be puffy and red and for my boys to know that their mum had a problem.

Why couldn't I ask for help? Why was I so stubborn? I could have asked for help and someone would have helped me, but I was too proud. I had no one to talk to about these issues because everyone assumed that I was OK. Nobody asked me what my life was really like. I was told that I was lucky. People said that life had been so good for me. Nobody asked, 'How do you cope with facial recognition issues?' or 'How do you find it when you go grocery shopping?' or 'Do you need a hand with anything?' I had fooled everyone but myself.

Life doesn't always go the way we'd like it to. At this time, our business was hugely affected by a very large debtor, and we had to take legal action. This was a very stressful time for us. We were running our business, driving the kids to and from school and sport, and there were business meetings to attend. One thing that brightened our day was a big red quarry truck. When the boys and I first saw this truck, the owner had a sign saying 'Baby Maker' on the bonnet. My son said that the truck driver must have a sense of humour and we should wave. OK, let's do it! We passed this truck, now known as 'our truck', once to three times a day and we waved every time. The boys would giggle in the back seat. We noticed one day that the owner had taken off the sign, but we could tell his truck from all the others a mile away, and we all still waved. It got to the point where my hand would go up to wave automatically when I saw 'our truck'.

One afternoon I drove into town alone, with the world on my shoulders – it had been one of my worst days. Something caught my

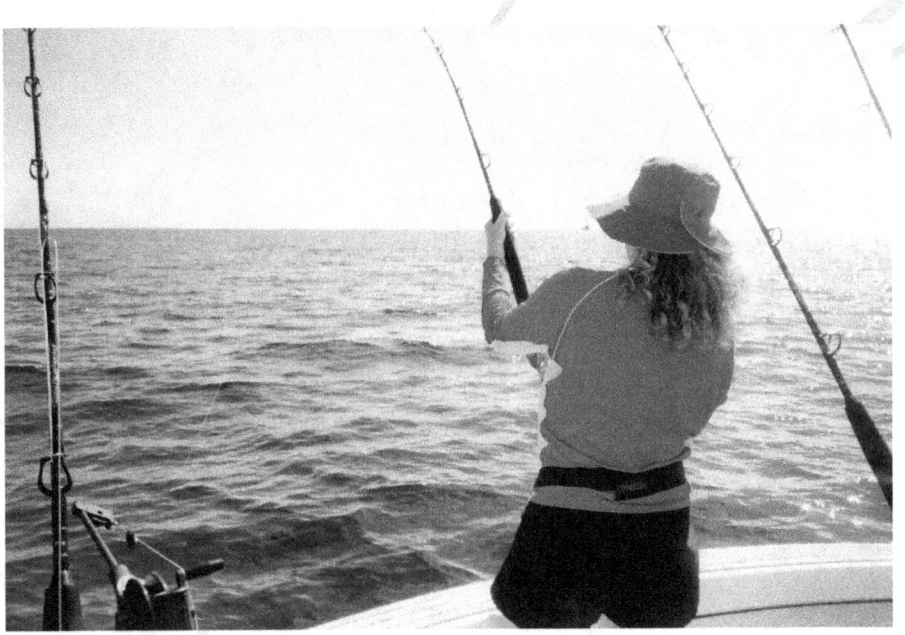
A new adventure – billfishing out on the open sea

eye, and as I looked up, there was 'our truck' and there was the driver waving at me with both hands and a big smile. I wished he had seen the smile that appeared on my face and seen all of the worries of the world slide off of my shoulders. I sent out a huge thank you to a man we never met in person for making such a difference in my life.

In the lead-up to the state election I spoke in front of over 300 professionals at a health forum. What did I speak about? Mental health, which was something close to my heart. The media interviewed me many times, and because of the speaking course I had done, I only had to remember three topics in relation to mental health. These were:

1. The past
2. Where we are now
3. What we are doing in the future

I also had to remember three things about each of these topics. Luckily, I was good with numbers, so remembering three things at a time sounded much easier than remembering a total number for the entire talk. I also found out that when a camera is staring you in the face but it's not live coverage, it is OK to stuff up because they will start the question and the camera again.

Running for parliament was a wonderful learning experience. I discovered that you don't have to believe everything they write about you in the paper. I have a thick skin now and I laughed at some of the comments that were made. I was also thankful for the fellow candidates who helped me through the campaign. One of them would call to warn me that I'd soon be getting a call from the ABC (because the ABC had just rung them to get their views on an issue). I would thank them and go off to do my research before receiving the call that asked me the same question. On the day of the election, I didn't win the seat – I had little funds and only weeks to prepare – but I did get enough votes to hold my head high and know that I had done my best.

However, we didn't stop there. We independents then stood in the local council election, which was held eight weeks later. We used our own money to run our campaigns. Friends and family helped out on both the local and state election days by handing out pamphlets and how-to-vote cards. I was number one on the ballot!

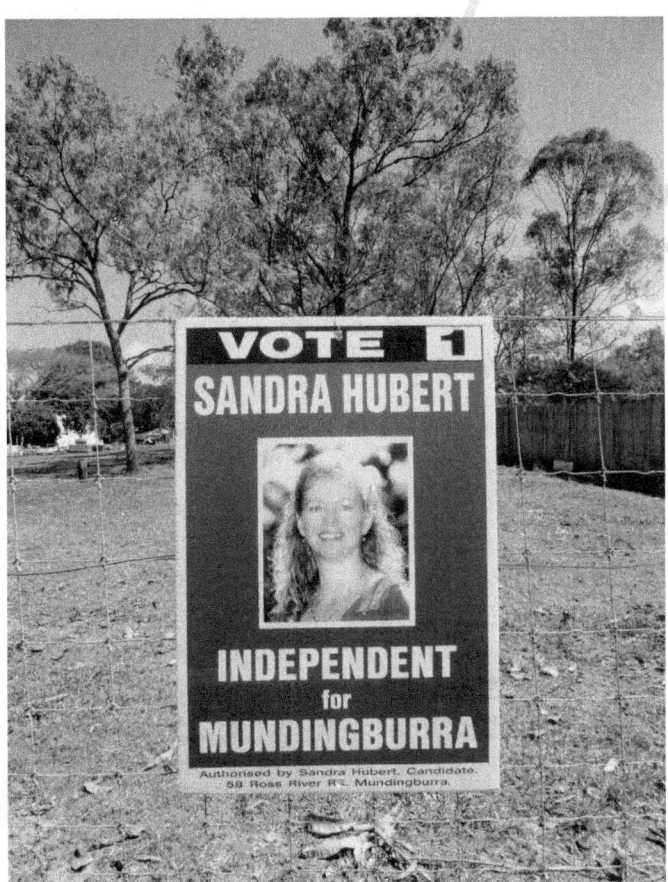
Corflute signage advertising my run for state government

Where does a girl go after all of this excitement? Well, this girl had to go to the doctor for a health issue – a specialist found a large grapefruit-sized cyst on one of my ovaries. When he wanted to book me in for surgery, I asked him to postpone it for a couple of weeks. He looked at me and asked why. I said, 'Well, I have a billfish tournament to go to and I want to tag a marlin.' He laughed and asked me to be careful. Luckily, I did tag and release a marlin, and it was such an adrenalin-pumping moment. I did everything right, with my 6kg line catching a marlin of approximately 30kg. Our deckhand didn't miss the tag, and the marlin was then released and swam away. Marlin are beautiful and graceful when jumping so high out of the water. The tags help scientists to understand the movements of these fish and you are notified if your marlin is caught again anywhere in the world. My cyst didn't burst while on the trip, and the keyhole surgery was a success because the cyst was only full of fluid. Who said a woman can't do everything?

I was too serious about life most of the time and I kept making higher goals for myself. I decided to remember where I started my recovery journey, to put structure into my day and to be able to laugh at myself. I enrolled in a shiatsu massage course and struggled with remembering the names of all of the muscles and bones in our body. I didn't have a problem with the practical exam but after the theory exam I phoned Roland, crying, thinking that I had failed drastically. I drove down the Strand, pulled over, looked out at the ocean and wrote down that I was stupid, and that I was dumb because I couldn't remember anything ... my list went on and on. I had to eat those words later because when my results arrived, I had received a high distinction, with 96%. How could I have thought so badly of myself? Roland hugged me and I cried. I was so sure that I had *failed* the theory test, and this showed me that I didn't have faith in myself.

Family is everything to me, and one day I saw a flyer from the boys' school advertising a group that helped you to adopt a grandparent. The 'grandparents' were people living in aged-care homes whom you could visit and include in your family. My parents didn't live locally, so I rang the group and nominated our family. They matched us with a lady called Julieanne. When I walked into the home's recreation room, which was full of aged people, I showed my letter to the staff and they took me over to Julieanne. However, I was confused. Julieanne was only 33 years of age. I discovered that

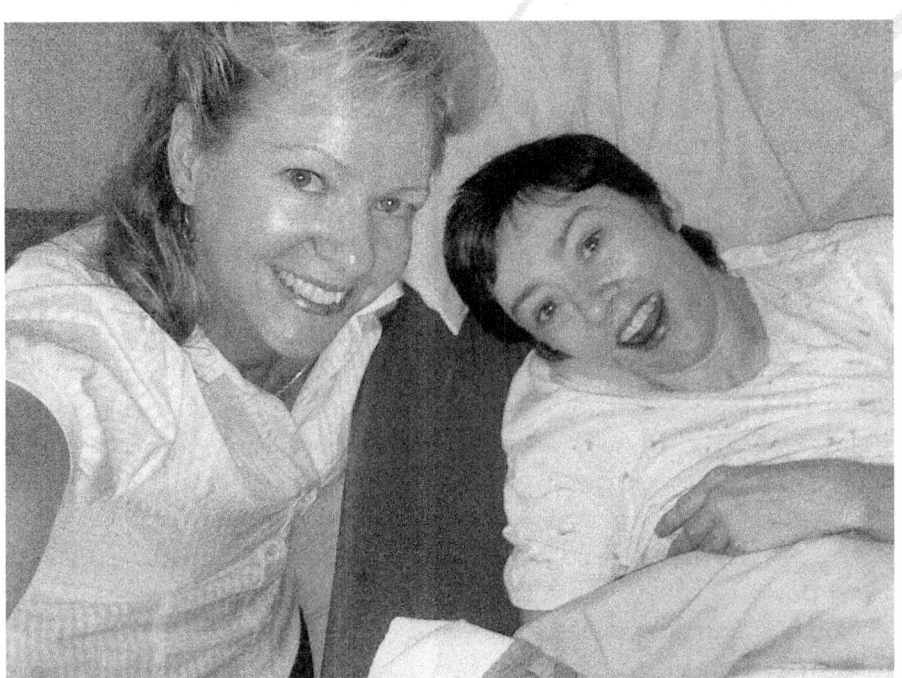
I loved spending time with Julieanne

she had Huntington's disease. It wasn't what I was expecting, but I believe that things happen for a reason and the friendship that developed between us over the years was so special.

When I walked into Julieanne's room every Tuesday afternoon, I often had the world on my shoulders and a mind full of problems. When I left her room, I realised that I didn't have a problem. You see, I could walk, I could pick up a photo of my son and kiss it. It broke my heart that I couldn't fix Julieanne's problems but I was also blessed to be able to brighten her day and her life. I asked her if I could take the photo that she had of her son (a photo that she wasn't able to pick up) and return it the next day. She said that I could. I had first thought that I would enlarge the photo but then thought better of it and instead printed it on a pillowcase so that Julieanne could move her head and kiss her son any time she wanted.

Julieanne helped me so much to understand myself. Once I pushed her in her wheelchair through the garden and we laughed when the sprinklers came on. Luckily the gardener heard us and quickly turned them off. We fed the turtles in the creek at the park and I read her stories. Her favourite song was 'Old MacDonald Had a Farm'. Julieanne always asked me to make the hardest animal noises and I did my best to make them. I would stay at mealtimes to feed her. She was given puréed food that didn't look appetising, so I would pretend that she was having something delicious. 'Tonight, we are having roast lamb with rosemary leaves, along with roast potato, pumpkin and carrot.' I would describe the tastes for her as she ate. She would smile and eat her meal.

When her sister passed away from the same disease, I held Julieanne and let her sob for as long as she needed to. Her family knew that she was being comforted as they grieved together. Seven years later, as Julieanne lay in palliative care, we could still communicate by blinking. One blink for no. Two blinks for yes and multiple blinks for 'I'll not tell you.' She would giggle at this and give me multiple blinks and I would smile with her. The staff told me that Julieanne was always better on the days when I visited. I didn't tell them, but so was I, and I treasured our times together. I knew that I'd receive a phone call soon from her dad to give me the sad news. When it came, I did my best to be strong. I am grateful to have those wonderful memories.

Chapter 26

In 2004, it was time for my 10-year check-up with Dr R, my neurologist. When I walked into his room, he looked over to me, smiled and held open his arms. He said, 'I still can't believe you are here. You have done so well.' This was such a profound statement from a man who sees so many people. (Later, in 2015, I asked Dr R for some information and his reply was, 'I can easily recall the details of your presentation and treatment back in 1994.' By then it had been 21 years since my injury, and it helped me to realise how far I had come and that I should not be so hard on myself. I needed to accept that I was so lucky to have survived my injury.)

My facial neuralgia, from the 1998 whiplash incident, had been ongoing. It was upsetting me so much that we decided to get legal advice. I wanted it to be documented that my condition was real. Luckily, because of my medical history, we had proof from before and after the incident – so, yes, I had a case. My lawyer was very understanding and helpful. I wanted for it to be documented and for it to be recognised that an injury had occurred. I also wanted all medical and legal expenses to be paid. We started the long legal process, a process that helped me to cope with the injury and to know that I had stood up for myself. The latter was something that I had had problems doing in the past.

The date for my case's mediation arrived and it was to be held in Brisbane. This meant two flights, a hotel stay and transport to and from the venue, as well as the mediation itself. For someone who is scared of flying and relies on her husband to accompany her to new things, it was a big step and one that I wanted to make. My dear friend's husband often had to go to Brisbane for work and he used a limo service while there. They gave me the name and number of this limo service and told me that they had told the owner to look after me. It helped me to know that I didn't have to wave down a taxi and hope that I got to my hotel. A driver called Brendan would be coming to pick me up at the airport. The limo service had all of my travel times booked, including travel to and from the courthouse. I also booked into the same hotel that we had stayed in when going to see concerts and shows, so it was familiar to me.

I found a dress to wear to court, which helped me to feel confident. My lawyer and barrister would be meeting me at the courthouse. I got off the plane and descended the airport escalator. I saw Brendan holding a sign with my name on it and it made me feel like a movie star. We walked over to retrieve my luggage and while we waited for my bag to come around the carousel, Brendan asked what colour my bag was. He then lifted it off the carousel for me. At no time did I have to carry it! Brendan took me to my hotel (carrying the bag to my room) and let me know when the limo would be arriving in the morning and who would be driving it. That night I was a bit nervous, so I read my notes and prepared for the morning. The next day, the limo arrived and off we went.

At mediation, we reach an agreement. Both sides were very thoughtful and understanding. My injury had been recognised, and it was now on record that it occurred because of a certain incident. I had to live with the pain but at least I had done what I could to have it acknowledged. It was real.

As we left the court, I told my barrister that I had to use my phone to make a call to my driver. On the call, I said, 'Hi, it's Sandy and I'm ready to be picked up. What colour is the car? What does he look like? Thank you.' My barrister and lawyer look at me quizzically and one asked, 'Why did you ask what colour the car was and what the guy looks like?' I smiled and replied, in a matter-of-fact way, that I wanted to know these details because a limo was coming to pick me up. As if on cue, a limo pulled up and the driver got out. He welcomed me as he opened the door, and I hopped into the car. The looks on the barrister's and lawyer's faces were classic, and they slightly shook their heads. I could imagine them thinking,

CHAPTER 26

'Who did we just represent? Is she a celebrity? Our clients don't usually get picked up by limos!' As they say, it's not what you know; it's who you know. I thanked my friend and her husband for making something that could have been so stressful into such a wonderful memory for me.

By this time, it had been 11 years since my illness, and Roland and I had achieved so much. It felt as though many pieces of my life had mended back together, and I liked that most people couldn't tell that I had a brain injury. Roland and I loved working together but we discussed my desire to work for an employer who wouldn't make allowances for my injury. Perhaps a new employer didn't even need to know that I had an injury. I was a bit stressed about going for a job interview after so many years, but I found an ad for a role that was perfect for me. I interviewed for the position of management accountant with a large company. The accountant/tax agent and the owner interviewed me. It had 11 businesses under a partnership, as well as three companies, and the businesses were diverse – agriculture, wholesale, retail, property and transport. It also had multiple locations in New South Wales and Queensland. During the interview I felt that the job was already mine, and I couldn't wait to start.

I landed the job, and jumped in with two feet – to land neck-deep in paperwork! However, this was fine because I was in my element. I found my way around the 11 businesses, became familiar with the three bank accounts and balanced all the inter-company loans. Soon I had everything in order, but I did go through many cups of coffee. One day the office staff came up to my office on the mezzanine floor to check on me. Why? I hadn't come down for a coffee and they hadn't heard my chair move. Well, I was doing a superannuation audit and I had multiple lever-arch folders open and was unable to move without dropping them. It was lovely to know that they cared!

I was surprised that budgets and forecasts hadn't been created, and I was told that it had been too hard to do. Oh, you should never tell me that because if you want it done, I can do it! So, I did. I didn't know the first thing about farming multiple types of fruits and vegetables, or about growing cane, but I made it my job to find out. I also worked with previous financial documentation and talked with managers and the owner until I had a full understanding of the needs of the businesses. I created a set of budgets and forecasts for all of the businesses, including a set for the entire business. I set these up to be live documents, which meant that if you changed one figure, all connecting figures automatically adjusted in the relevant areas. My boss gave me a big smile – he knew that he could trust me to do my job well.

After this I worked on the trucking business, listing all of the trucks and vehicles and documenting their fuel consumption, tyre rotations, wheel-bearing maintenance and services. I spoke with my mechanic, and with a friend who has trucks, to find the best method to keep our trucks on the road. From my office I could tell, by my spreadsheet calculations, if a truck needed a service or if it was using too much fuel. This was helpful, because we didn't want them breaking down halfway across Australia. Our truck drivers were very helpful and gave me the information I needed each week. All I was doing was keeping them on the road. I really enjoyed the type of mental stimulation that this job provided.

In 2005, Roland had to take a business trip to Newcastle and the flight was going to have an overnight stay in Sydney. It was around the time of my birthday, so we decided to go together. I had been wanting to go to Sydney and visit the Opera House ever since I was a teenager. My girlfriend Susan had rung me from the steps of the Opera House in 1981 and I had promised her that when I got to Sydney one day, I would ring her. I was also excited because we were going to see a production of *The Lion King* that night.

While driving us straight from the airport to the Opera House, the taxi driver could see how excited I was. We chatted away while I took photos out of the window. I could see the Opera House entrance, and there were a lot of security guards there. I didn't realise that there wasn't usually that much security there, so I almost fell into a heap when we were stopped and told that there had been a security breach – because of that they were not letting cars park there.

I was within running distance of the place I had waited 24 years to get to. Our taxi driver looked at me in his rear-vision mirror and turned to ask security if he could drop off his passengers at the Opera House and then return in an hour to pick us up. Security didn't have any problems with people being there, so this proposal was fine by them. My head was racing. What? Leave my luggage in a taxi with someone I don't know who says they'll be back in an hour to pick

> *My boss gave me a big smile – he knew that he could trust me to do my job well.*

us up? Roland and I looked at each other and at the taxi driver. My shattered look was all they both needed to see – the driver drove us in and told us when he would return.

Holding hands, Roland and I walked up the Opera House stairs, and I quickly grabbed my phone so that I could call Susan. Roland smiled. I hoped and prayed that Susan would pick up the phone (we usually play phone tag). I was over the moon when she answered. 'Hi Sandy, how are you?' 'Oh, Susan, I'm standing on the steps of the Opera House and I had to ring you.' 'You remembered!' she replied. With tears in my eyes, I said, 'I made a promise to you. It may have taken me 24 years, but I'm here ringing you.' We chatted for a bit and she thanked me for remembering. Then Roland and I went around exploring the Opera House. After an hour, our taxi driver appeared, just as he had said he would, ready to take us to our hotel. It was a magical day and I thank this random taxi driver for making my dreams come true. The production of *The Lion King* was awesome, and it was one of the best birthdays I have had.

After the elections, we continued meeting with Bob Katter to work out more policies and plans. One day, Bob picked me up from my workplace on his way to one of those meetings. You should have seen my co-workers – they couldn't believe it when Bob popped in and chatted to them all. It was Bob who got the surprise when I hopped in the car and realised that I knew the limo driver. Perhaps I do know a lot of people!

At another time, Mark Taylor the cricketer was in the news. Coincidentally, I have a friend with the same name. My friend Mark rang me at work one day and the staff were in a tizzy because Mark Taylor had rung for me. I had to let them know that it wasn't the famous Mark who was in the news. There was also the time my co-workers told me that they saw me on the national news. The story was about the billfish tournament, and our team was dressed as the Olympic synchronised drinking team. The TV crew I had worked with for the business awards had seen me on the boat, so they came over to interview us. If you'd like to learn the moves of the synchronised drinking team, simply stand your team in a line with you all wearing your swim gear, with sheets wrapped around you and a crown of leaves in your hair. Hold your drinks in your right hand and all together do a 360-degree spin-turn to your right. Then take a sip of your drink. Or something like that. There is a serious side and a

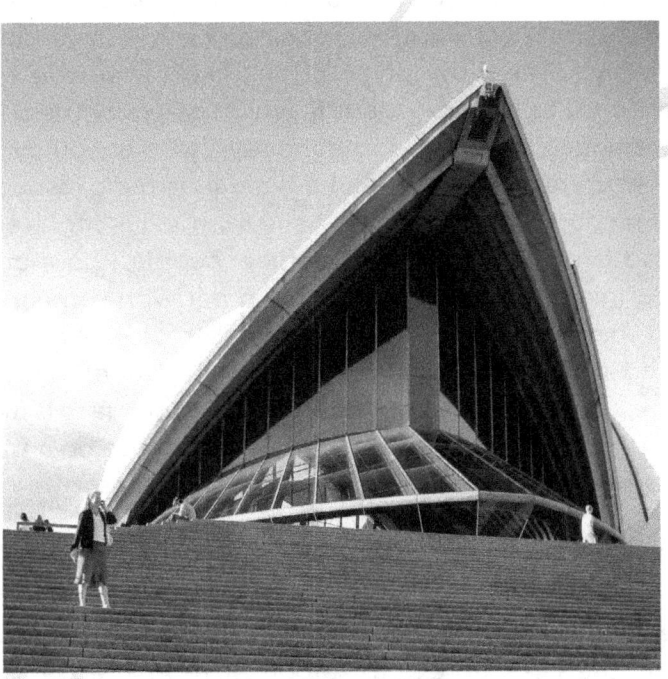

Calling Susan from the steps of the Opera House!

fun side to me. I have learned to laugh at myself and not to take life so seriously.

I was in a job where I met many people, but my facial recognition issues made it hard for me to remember everyone when I saw them outside of a work context. I found it difficult to put a name to a face when in a different setting. I had a good psychologist who taught me mindfulness and to be aware of my body's reactions. When you see someone you know, you may smile or wave if it's a friend, or your back may straighten (or you may automatically extend your hand for a handshake) if it's a business acquaintance. You may clench your teeth when you see a person you don't like. I used this automatic bodily response to help me identify which category the person was from. Take notice next time someone says hello to you. Be aware of how your body responds – we all have an automatic response.

Facial recognition is still a big issue for me. I recognise all of my friends and family, but when I meet new people, I have problems. I have a technique I use when I have to meet with someone: I arrive early, and then they have to look for me. I also use Facebook to find their photo, and I save the photo with their number in my phone. I look at the photo before our meeting so that their face is fresh in my memory. I'm very hard on myself and don't want to be embarrassed by not recognising someone, or to have that person realise that I have a problem. This is why I love business meetings and functions; we usually all wear name badges.

One day I raced from my car to the door of a function centre, to attend a Townsville Business Women's Network event. I arrived at the door at the same time as a six-foot-tall red-haired lady. We both stopped and looked at each other. I smiled and said, 'I love meeting tall ladies,' and she replied with, 'So do I. Why don't we sit together?' This was the start of a wonderful friendship with Jennifer. She ran a social women's group called WOW, which stands for Women of Worth (or, later in the day, Women on Wine). Our husbands lovingly called it Witches on Wine, but we disagreed, with a smile. The group still runs, with us meeting for lunch on the first Sunday of each month. It's not about business; it's about people, laughter, friendship and feeling included. For those two hours we talk, laugh, share our concerns and celebrate our achievements, and when lunch is over husbands can join us or we go our separate ways.

CHAPTER 26

Growing up, I always had more male friends than female friends so it is wonderful now to have so many girlfriends. Nobody judges anyone. Every month we write in the WOW book and Jennifer takes photos of us to put in the book (we see comments such as, 'Lovely lunch with a great group of women', 'My first lunch and I so look forward to seeing you all again next time' and 'Great food, great friends and fun times'). We are up to book three now and it is fabulous to flick through the pages, which feature all of our lunches and events from over the years. I love reading the comments and reminiscing. To think that my WOW friendships all started from one chance meeting with a lady who has become a lifelong friend. Have you ever met someone by chance and it has made a positive difference in your life? Actually, I have to stop writing for a moment because I'm about to head off to another WOW lunch. I won't have to stress about facial recognition because all I'll have to do is look for a six-foot redhead, and we all wear name tags. There can be between six and over 30 ladies at lunch, and new ladies are always welcome. Yes, we are always the loudest table at the restaurant! I'll be home in time to get ready for our weekly Sunday family dinner.

———————

Chapter 27

The year 2006 was another busy one for me. I saw an advertisement for the AGM of Wee Care, and it reminded me of a promise I had made nearly 30 years before, when I was a Girl Guide. To earn one of my badges, I used to volunteer at Wee Care, which looked after children needing foster care or immediate care. I loved helping to look after these children and I had promised that one day I would come back and help. The other reason that the ad caught my attention was the fact that a lady called Mary Gibson was the chairperson, and I had worked for Mary before, doing tax returns. I rang Mary, and she said that she would be honoured to have me join the Wee Care management committee. It was wonderful to be able to help these children again and be part of such an important community-based group in our town. Later, in 2012 and 2013, I became the chairperson and it was such an honour to do that work. The organisation is now known as Althea Projects Incorporated (it was renamed in 2013 to honour the ladies who started the organisation in the early 1970s, in the aftermath of cyclone Althea), which saw the need for crisis care for children. It is a privilege to have helped so many families and children.

I looked for a local group that supported people with brain injury, but I hadn't yet found one. So, in 2006 I joined the committee of Mental Illness Fellowship North Queensland. It was as close as I had found to a group that dealt with brain injury, and through it I hoped to discover more about the brain and recovery.

Later that year, I was asked to participate in the Greater North Queensland Leadership Summit. This involved 30 managers from across Queensland coming together to write a white paper (a report) on rural and remote management issues. It was meant to be a think tank to build local leadership capability, job skills and job retention, and innovation. It was held over two days at Mission Beach. It was a wonderful experience to be part of those workshops and to meet such a diverse group of managers. We understood that large cities had access to more than our rural areas, but we wanted to do what we could to bring these issues forward and provide sufficient opportunities and challenges for everyone.

On one occasion, I was lucky to be in Brisbane on my mum's birthday, so I surprised her. I knocked on her door with a bunch of flowers in one hand and a cold bottle of Champagne in the other. She squealed with joy and didn't know what to do first – hug me or take the flowers or the bottle of Champagne! She was so excited. We had a wonderful day together, not realising that 12 months later she would arrive at my front door, wrapping her fragile arms around me, needing me to care for her due to the onset of dementia. My mum had looked after me and now it was my turn to look after her.

In all my years of organising business and management awards, I had never considered being a judge. However, in 2007 I was asked by the AIM if I would be a judge for its management awards. I accepted this challenge. I then thought it would be a good idea to answer the judging questions for myself, to get a better understanding of what was expected. The questions were enlightening. I believe that everyone should ask themselves similar questions, so that they can realise what they have achieved in their work life. Do this with me. Write down what is your management approach, and what type of manager you try to be. What are your skills and where do you see yourself in five or 10 years? What are your personal and business achievements? We don't often stop to see where we have been and to acknowledge our achievements. I'd like you to take a moment to write down yours. Over the course of my recovery, I have forgotten many of my achievements, so I have started to write them down. It is so easy to write the negatives, but we need to write down our achievements, too.

I enjoyed being a judge in 2007 and 2008, and seeing the achievements of so many people. Wearing my other hat, in my role as

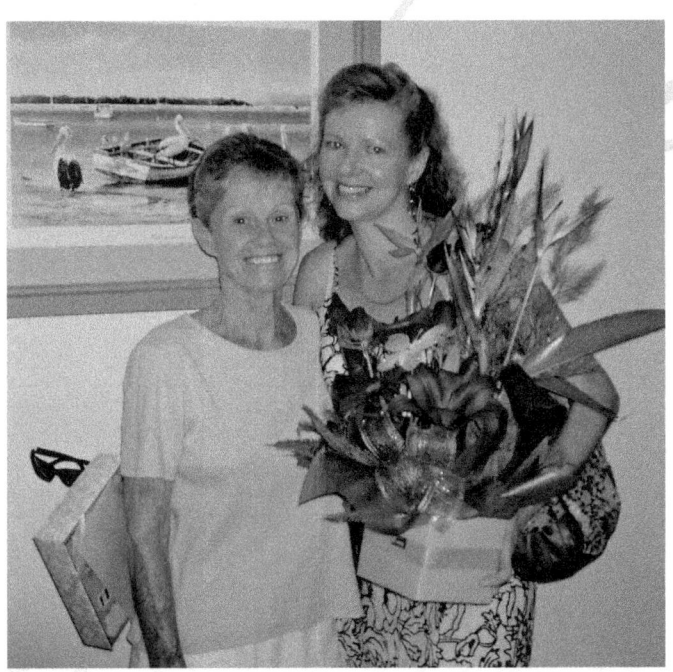
Surprising Mum on her birthday, November 2006

president of the Past Students' Association, I also met lovely students who applied for the Past Students' Scholarship. Interviewing those teenagers and hearing what they had accomplished in their life so far, and what their goals and career choices were, was a truly humbling experience.

Chapter 28

In 2007 Jaiden started high school. Hadn't time passed so quickly? Our two older boys were working in Townsville and living with their mates. But with boys being boys, they often came back home for a feed. As I mentioned earlier, my mum was staying with us and she was in the early stages of dementia. Our doctor was very supportive and helping me to adjust to these demands. I was working full time and still doing all of my volunteer and committee work. Yes, it was a long list – I was on the management committees of Wee Care and Mental Illness Fellowship North Queensland, and on the executive committee of the AIM. I was also the president of The Cathedral School Past Students' Association, treasurer of the Monique Robinson Trust Fund, and a volunteer at the Good Shepherd Hospice where I visited Julieanne. Oh, and I was also a soroptimist, on the organisation's executive and health committee. It's no wonder that I received a certificate of appreciation for Australian volunteers from the prime minister of Australia at the time, John Howard. However, I didn't do it for the recognition – I just loved the work that I was doing. Luckily, meetings were held on different nights, and lunches were on different days, so I could attend them all. Being organised, I had a briefcase for each board and committee and only one diary.

We continued to enjoy our camping holidays, and I seemed to cope even though I could become a bit disorientated. When we went sightseeing, Roland or my friend Glenda would usually stay close to me so that I didn't get lost. However, nobody thought that

I had any problems when we stayed at a caravan park. I had my coping strategies. When it came to using the laundry facilities, I waited until someone else went to use them and I would tag along so that I wouldn't get lost. I would forget which machine I had used, so to remedy this I either stayed with the machine or left something on top of the machine. When I hung up the clothes on the line, I used orange pegs so that I could find our clothes again later. This was all very stressful for me, and I noticed that I felt a little ill after our holidays and had tummy trouble.

The issues came to light one holiday when our caravan was on an en suite site. Roland noticed that I did all of my washing by hand in the basin of the en suite, and I didn't have any tummy troubles. It dawned on us that even though I may have needed to go to the toilet, I would wait until someone went to the amenities block and I would go with them. I was too embarrassed to ask someone to take me, so I would wait all day, if needed. That was why I was having tummy troubles. Why didn't I ask someone, or tell Roland? Well, I had tried to rely on the old 'I'll do it myself' approach, but I should have asked for help – I just didn't know how. As soon as we got home, Roland set about finding a caravan that had an en suite and a washing machine so that I could relax and enjoy our holidays. On the following Easter holidays, we christened our new second-hand caravan, which featured an en suite and laundry, and it was wonderful. We still have that caravan (affectionately called Yakabit because Roland likes to yak a bit) and she has been a fabulous addition to our family.

Later that year, Roland received an unexpected call. It was from a company that was building a shopping centre in Fiji. Its supervisor had quit, and management wanted Roland to start with the company immediately. It was like a whirlwind having to get his passport and work visas in time for him to fly out. Fiji had been a special place for Roland's parents because they had worked and lived there in the '50s. It was also a sad place because their third child, a boy, had only lived one day and had been buried in Fiji in an unmarked grave. The last thing Roland said to us as he boarded that plane was, 'I'm going to find my brother.'

The Fijians accepted Roland with open arms and when they found out about his brother, they all pitched in to help him. Roland spoke with the security guard at the prison where all records were kept, and they found out that their fathers had worked together.

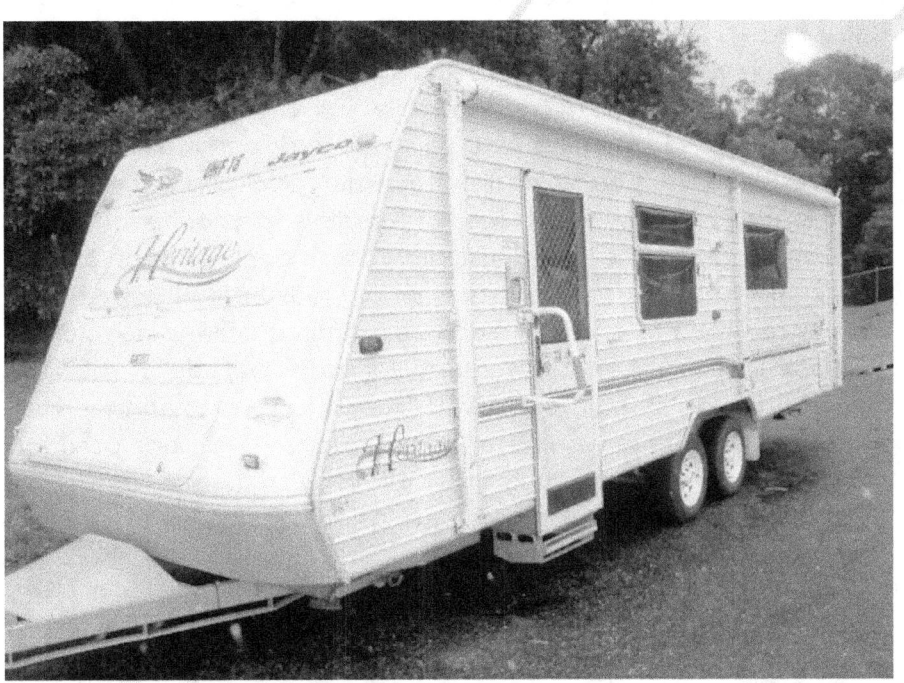
Yakabit, the caravan that has hosted so many holiday memories

With this connection, Roland searched the old paper records from 1955 and found the entry for Ronald, Roland's brother. Now they knew where he was buried. They both got into a taxi and headed there. When they arrived at the cemetery, the security guard and the taxi driver got out with Roland because they wanted to help find Ronald's grave. On 11 November 2007, we received the best gift of all – a text message that read, 'I've found my brother's grave. It's raining and I'll come back with flowers for Mum' (meaning that he would go back to the grave and place flowers there on behalf of his mum and dad). He had phoned his mum and she had started crying straight away, so he asked me to go over and see his parents. I drove straight over and we hugged and cried together.

We organised for a plaque to be made and sent from Townsville, and the Fijians helped Roland build a memorial plinth for it. I sent photos and personal items to go in Ronald's memorial, so that we were all with him. The Fijians also did a traditional dance and prayer for Ronald, and they said that they would look after his grave when Roland returned to Australia. Such beautiful and caring people.

Back in Townsville, I was caring for Mum outside of my work hours (although she did come with me to functions) and we were all coping. We had a wonderful neighbourhood – on one occasion, mum went for a wander and I was all ready to go in search of her when a car pulled up with my mum inside. One of Jaiden's friends had seen my mum walking and had said to their mum, 'Hey that's Jaiden's nanna.' They picked her up and drove her home. It was a real awakening for what we would need to do to care for my mum. I took her almost everywhere I could with me; otherwise, my elderly neighbours Rob and Val looked after her for me. They would invite her over for a cuppa and give me the wink that mum would be fine with them. They were a beautiful couple.

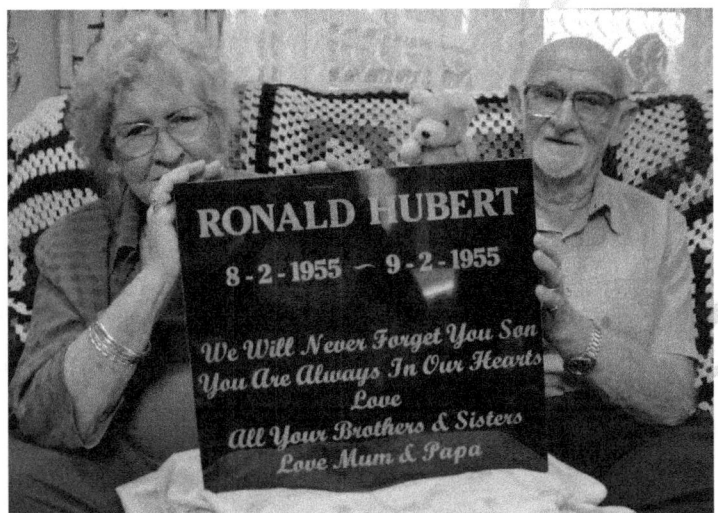

Roland's parents, holding the beautiful plaque that honoured their baby son

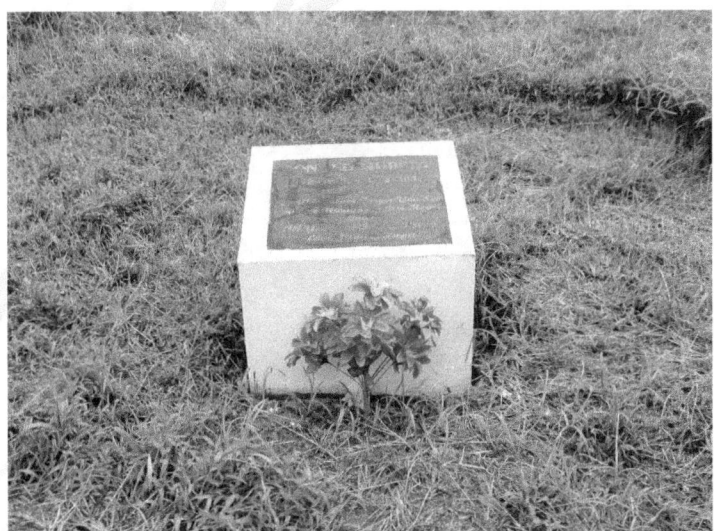

Ronald's memorial in Fiji

Chapter 29

In 2008 it was a surprise when I received a letter from the mayor of Thuringowa, letting me know that I had been nominated for the Spirit of Thuringowa Award for my contribution to the Thuringowa community. At the ceremony, mayor Les Tyrell said that he would really enjoy handing out the next award to a true ambassador for our city ... Mrs Sandra Hubert! The mayor had sat beside me in meetings with the Thuringowa Chamber of Commerce; he had witnessed my role with the Thuringowa Business Awards; and he had read about all of the other volunteer work that I had done in the community. It was an honour to stand beside him. He not only shook my hand; he also gave me a hug. This certificate hangs proudly on the wall in my office.

A few months later, I received a letter from the Townsville Business Women's Network saying that I had been nominated for the Corporate Business Woman of the Year award. I had no idea who nominated me but I was very excited and nervous. I had to accept the nomination and complete the entry form. Then I attended a 'Meet the Finalist' function, where I met all the award nominees. I can't remember how many finalists they chose in each category, but when they called out my name, I was ecstatic. I hugged a friend who was nominated but not chosen as a finalist (it surprised me that she wasn't a finalist, because I knew how hard she had worked). It seemed that all of a sudden, I was receiving acknowledgment for the work I had done. I was so busy doing the work that it hadn't occurred to me to receive recognition. It's just me giving to other people.

My job also required a lot of legal work, which took up a lot of my time. Our lawyers even gave me an office for a couple of days so that I could categorise and document all of the evidence. The secretary made sure that I had enough coffee, and the lawyers gave me a wave or a nod. They showed me the type of respect that I didn't show to myself. It helped me accept myself and to see myself as others do. I suppose I assumed that people saw me with a huge mark on my head that tells people, 'I'm dumb and have a brain injury.' Yet, sitting in that office with people for whom I have a lot of respect, and who showed me respect, made me realise how hard I was on myself.

With the awards coming up, we had tickets for ourselves and for our friends. I had my new ballgown ready. I received an email letting me know that they wanted to organise a time to come to my workplace to video it for the presentations. It seemed that I was more excited about this than my co-workers. Our warehouse was usually so busy with people, forklifts, trucks and produce everywhere. The office staff would be at their desks or walking around. Usually, I could count between 10 and 30 people. However, the television crew turned up and – blink – not a soul to be seen. The crew chatted to me for a while and videoed me in my office. This may have relaxed the staff a little, because we managed to film some of them working in the warehouse and my boss driving the forklift.

Awards night came, and the photographer was none other than the *Townsville Bulletin*'s photographer, who had taken my photo many times. So Roland and I posed for what we felt was the photo of the year, which they printed in the newspaper.

Nobody but three of the people at my table knew anything about my brain injury and my journey of survival and recovery. When it came time to announce the winner of my award, they told us that they would call out the top three finalists, in no particular order, and they were to come to the stage. My nerves were on edge, and I wondered what I would say if I won. Drum roll. Sandra Hubert, please come to the stage! There I was, standing with flowers and a finalist certificate in my hand, next to the other two finalists. My name wasn't called out as the winner, but by standing on that stage in front of all those people, I already was a winner. I didn't need a trophy because my husband, family and friends were proud of me.

One of the judges came over to me during the evening and told me that I should have won. It was a reminder to me of how

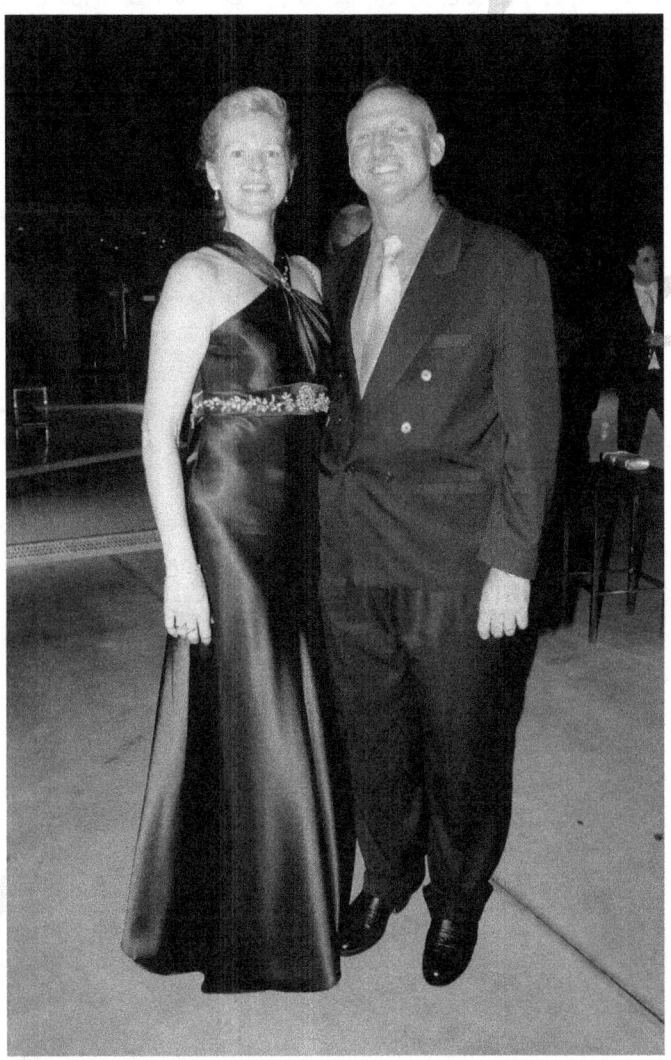

Roland and I at the awards night where I was nominated for Corporate Business Woman of the Year

well I covered my disabilities so that nobody could see them. At the interview for the awards, I didn't tell the panel of my brain injury and I didn't ask for any allowances. When they asked me the questions, I didn't give myself enough time to process and answer them. My mind went blank and I didn't explain to them that I needed time to process information, to understand what was asked of me and to formulate an answer. When answering on paper it was so easy because I could look up my trusty dictionary, look into my thesaurus for similar words and write, check and rewrite my answer. When writing this book, I realised that I wasn't sharing the entire reality of my life on these pages – I was minimising the problems I encountered in life after my brain injury, and made it sound as though my life was happy and easy. At night, my mind would go over what I had written for this book, and I would then remember the strength that I had needed to get up each day, the times I had wanted to give up, the days I had cried, the willpower I had needed to show up for work, and the strategies I had put in place to be just like everyone else. I was still in the habit of hiding my reality.

When my photo from the awards night appeared in the newspaper, along with a lovely write-up about the finalists and the winners, it solidified the impression to others that I am OK and that I am living a full, successful and happy life. Why would I want anyone to think otherwise?

This was also the year that our second-born turned 21. Kyle and his beautiful girlfriend Lauren had flown back to Townsville from Perth for his birthday, and her birthday was three weeks after his. So, of course, I was to hold a double 21st birthday party for them. We scheduled it for Saturday 4 October. However, things changed quickly. On the Thursday, Kyle was going to take Lauren out to dinner. While she was getting ready, he asked me if he could borrow a suit from his dad. He then told me that he wanted to propose to Lauren as a surprise, before they went out to dinner. Well, we found a suit that fitted, I threw a bottle of Champagne in the freezer and I raced into the garden to cut some roses.

Picture this: Roland and I are sitting on the lounge with our cameras ready and our backs to the hallway. Kyle is in a suit, holding the box containing a beautiful ring he'd had made, and also holding a rose. We are all trying to act 'normal'. Out walks Lauren, and Kyle goes down on his bended knee and proposes. Lauren

CHAPTER 29

says yes. Kyle places the ring on her finger and she jumps into his arms. Roland and I are there to take precious photos of this awesome moment and then to hug the happy couple. Oh, wow, such a special moment! We reminded them to ring Lauren's parents because we knew how excited Tracy and Dave would be. The next 24 hours were spent with me changing the announcement in the newspaper (from a double 21st birthday to an engagement), ringing everyone to announce that it was to be a double 21st birthday party *and* an engagement party, as well as re-doing the cake, decorations and photos.

Roland's oldest brother, Tyrone, had been unwell for some time, and on the morning of the party we received news that his condition was worsening and that he may not have much longer to live. His parents and sister flew from Townsville to Brisbane, and he died just before the party started. We decided to go ahead with the party – all families deal with problems differently, and we wanted the party to commemorate the loss of a wonderful uncle, son, brother, husband and father. Our son and his beautiful fiancée took all of this in their stride as we came together to celebrate their 21st birthdays and the joy of their engagement and to honour the loss of a loved one.

Chapter 30

The year 2009 started with sadness after the loss of Tyrone, and sadness struck again when my awesome girlfriend Robyn had the fight of her life with cancer. On one particular day, I had presented PSA scholarships on stage, in front of the entire school and parents. I had come a long way from being an anxious young schoolgirl who found it hard to talk in front of her 24 fellow students. On this day there were over 700 people in attendance ... and my speech was easy compared to the hour-long phone call that I had later with Robyn.

She rang to say goodbye. We cried and reminisced about all the fun times we had had together and told each other how much we loved each other and what our friendship meant. We laughed about the time when Roland and I had come to Brisbane to visit. With Robyn being Robyn, she had yelled out to Roland (who was on his way to the toilet), 'Make sure you put the lid down!' Well, it was on the way home that Roland told me what he had done. Yes, he had put the toilet seat down but he had taken the seat *off* of the toilet and placed it on the floor. Roland and Robyn were always playing tricks on each other. We all laughed a lot when she rang to tell Roland off. His reply was, 'You told me to put the lid down, so I did.' My beautiful friend – who will always be 49 – is someone I will never forget. Love you, Robyn.

My way of coping with things is to do something practical. Around this time, my car was making noises and I suspected that it was to do with a CV joint. I contacted my mechanic, who confirmed my diagnosis. I asked him if he would assist me with changing the CV myself. A strange ask of a female, perhaps, but he liked the idea so he booked us in for a late afternoon and ordered the parts. Sitting on the floor of the garage – with grease up my arms as I removed the brakes, straightened the axle, and removed and replaced the CV joint – was great. My trusty mechanic offsider was there to lift the heavy wheel and tell me what steps I had to take. I did it myself and I was so proud that I could. I have to admit that the first feeling of grease on my hands was tough to cope with, but after that I didn't even think about it. It was another reminder of the things that I used to do before my injury.

To learn more about my brain and to help others with a disability, I attended a STEPS leader training program. STEPS is short for Skills to Enable People and CommunitieS. The course was excellent and it gave me skills that have helped me. It also made me aware of the importance of having short- and long-term goals, and of breaking down each step towards the achievement of those goals. I felt so comfortable being with people who have a disability. This was strange because I really didn't have a disability, but it made me realise all that I had achieved and that I wanted to help others strive for and achieve *their* goals. It's all about giving it a go and not letting other people tell you that you won't be able to do something.

I went in search of a brain injury social group and found one that enjoyed dinners every fortnight. Roland and I decided to join these dinners, and we made many new friends. Most of them had been in an accident or had a brain tumour and their injuries were more visible than mine. I was often mistaken for a carer or for the organiser of the event. This helped me to understand who I was and where I fitted into the world because I didn't have the problems of these guys. They became my friends and I felt very protective of them all, especially when people stared or were rude.

So, when the position of coordinator for the group came up, I put up my hand. We then started to call the group 'A.B.I. be in it'. We planned the year and I printed out a calendar of events that included dress-up dinners. We had a Mad Hatter's Tea Party at Easter, a Melbourne Cup celebration (including a sweep), and Halloween and Christmas, as well as a few events such as 'come as your favourite movie character'. These were fun nights because everyone loved

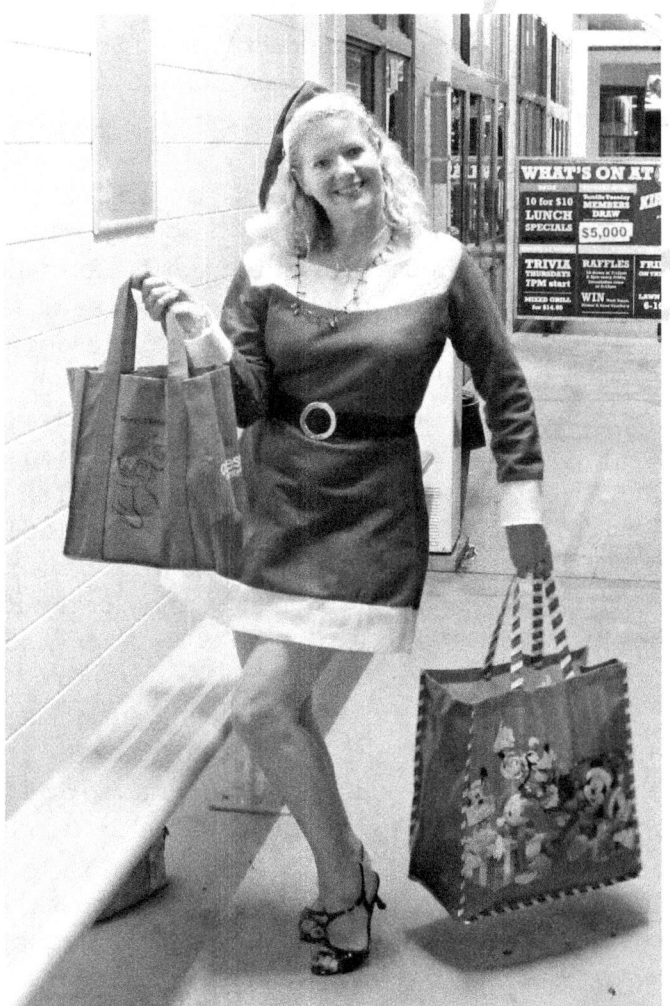

Sandra Clause, at your service

dressing up and enjoying themselves. One night we had karaoke with a difference, with everyone just singing whatever they wanted to the music. It was awesome. The restaurant staff were wonderful and made sure we either had our own room or a separate area. They treated our members with respect and let us make as much noise as they liked, and nobody minded. We had Secret Santa every year, with fun gifts, and I dressed up as Sandra Clause with Roland playing Santa. One year Roland turned up in a blown-up Santa suit, riding a reindeer. It was such fun.

In the early part of the year, I received a phone call from a young man who had been a previous employee of my workplace. The call seemed genuine because he wanted some information about his employment and, as the accountant, I was able to assist him. What I didn't realise was that it was the start of stalking. It started as an innocent phone call that led to him making many calls from different numbers, or sending me text messages. I had no idea how to stop them. I didn't know how to be rude and just hang up. 'I have to go now.' 'Why?' I didn't have an answer. This went on for months. I felt total fear, so I phoned my psychologist, Dr McDonald. He calmed me down and chatted with me for half an hour. He gave me coping techniques to use, as well as words to say the next time the stalker rang. I kept blocking the phone number the stalker used, but the numbers changed all the time. Anxiety hit me every time the phone rang. He never threatened me, but the calls were not acceptable. Nothing I said had stopped him, so I had to go to the police. This was scary, too, but I was developing PTSD and had to do something. I was even too scared to go to bed because that's when the nightmares would begin.

The police were very understanding and said that they would contact him and ask him to stop. They knew how to handle people such as these. I thanked them so much for believing me and helping me. Sometimes standing up for yourself is the hardest thing to do because you don't know how people will respond. The phone calls stopped, and then all I had to do was cope with my PTSD. This experience brought back the feelings I had when I was in the coma – the fear, the pain, the cold and the feeling of being lost. One of my psychologists helped me with mindfulness. I was able to focus on things other than what was in my mind. It helped to place me in the here and now. I practised breathing techniques to ease anxiety and

> *I feel for people who go through PTSD because it totally consumes you.*

to help me go to sleep. I laid on my bed in the daylight to prove that nothing happened to me if I laid on my bed. I feel for people who go through PTSD because it totally consumes you.

There were nights when I woke up with my heart pounding, and feeling so much fear that I wanted to run away – but I didn't because the thought of getting out of bed was also scary. Almost like hiding from a monster under the covers ... Then I'd toss and turn for two to three hours, trying to go back to sleep. Have you ever experienced this? 'Take a sleeping pill,' someone said. No. Why? Well, my body reacts differently to the way it does for most people, and it always has. For example, my skin doesn't go numb with a normal local anaesthetic; coffee helps put me to sleep; and even some of the strongest pain relief tablets don't have any effect on me – they don't even make me drowsy. From a very young age, I that found relaxation techniques and Reiki worked best. So, my worry about taking sleeping tablets was that my reaction to them was unknown; therefore, I was too fearful to try one.

Roland was with me every step of the way. Our lives had been very diversified (working in different careers, working together, working for ourselves, organising big events, racing, being involved in politics ...) but I was still trying to find out who I was and to feel part of the world. Roland had to cope with loving me, yet he also felt extremely hurt that I had nearly died. Without realising it, he had started to build a wall between us to protect his pain. This didn't help our marriage and we had to find someone to help us remove that wall and the pain he was feeling. Nobody warned us that this could happen. We wanted to be together, put the past behind us and be 'us' again.

We were different from the people we were when we met. I would hear a psychologist ask, 'Has your brain injury changed your personality?' My answer would be no, because the real me hasn't changed. The social barriers we often build up over time had gone for me, so I had become more like the person I had been as a teenager. I had to remind psychologists and doctors that everyone changes over time. At our 30-year school reunion, my classmates said that I hadn't changed a bit, whereas they had. Roland had changed, too. He had been beside me through everything and had coped in the best way that he could. To make our own personal statement of our love and commitment to each other, we decided to renew our vows

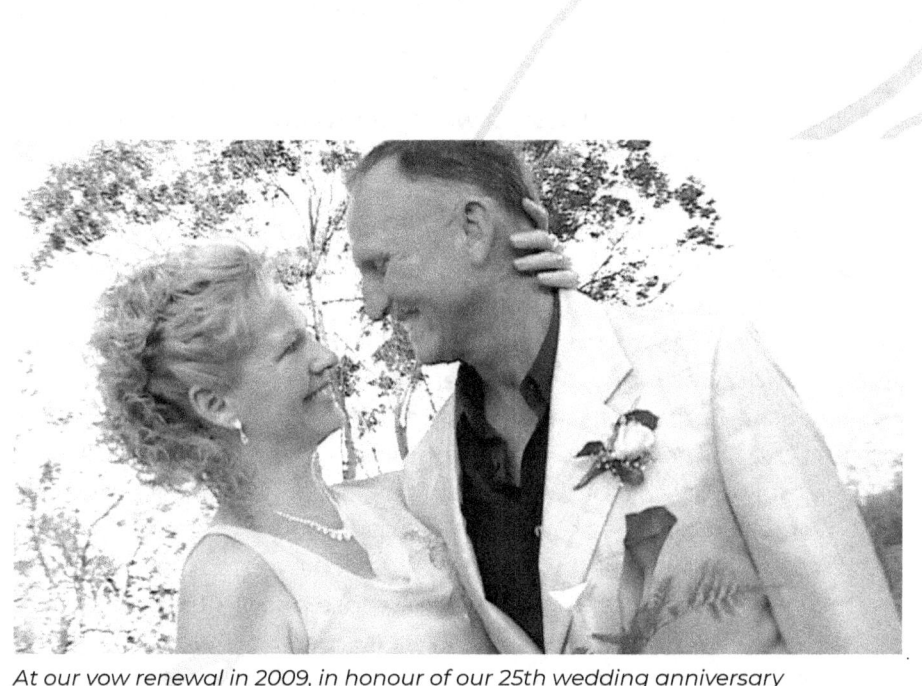
At our vow renewal in 2009, in honour of our 25th wedding anniversary

for our 25th wedding anniversary, in December 2009. We both loved the new people we had become and wanted to symbolise this in front of family and friends.

On our special day, everyone stood at Pipers Lookout (which overlooks our city) on Hervey Range, waiting for me to walk down the red carpet. I first walked over to the memorial of our dear friend's wife Jenny, who had tragically died, and placed flowers there. I then joined Roland and we let go of balloons that represented loved ones who had passed. It was a symbolic way of thanking the past, letting go of the pain and making a vow for our future together. So, with family and friends as witnesses, we renewed our vows. Afterwards, I had everyone choose a 'wish rock', make a wish and then throw the rock off the mountain. There were many giggles and much laughter and I hoped that their wishes would come true.

So much was happening at work at that time, and because my employer was involved in a forthcoming court case I was once again in the thick of legal representation. My learning curve was a straight line up and I was enjoying it. I spent many hours in meetings with lawyers and barristers alongside my employer, who relied on me to present the financial information required. At one meeting, a lawyer jokingly called me his barrister and I quickly looked at my employer, who reminded me that my pay rate wasn't going to change. We all had a giggle about this. It was a personal achievement for me to see that my work ethic was appreciated by those people. In the business world, I excelled and it was still only in my personal world that I felt awkward and misplaced. This was crazy, really, because I was such a social person. I just felt that something was missing, and that it had to do with facial recognition and short-term memory issues. I was the best friend with whom your secrets would be safe because I would forget that you had told them to me. On the other hand, I would forget the things that you told me that I *should* remember, and I would ask you about them. That was what upset me because I knew that I wasn't the person I used to be. However, I would remember your birthday – my propensity for numbers helped me!

I continued trying to understand my body and its reactions. One day in my office I felt panicky, claustrophobic feelings that I couldn't explain. I loved my office and felt safe there. Someone came into my office and straight away said, 'Oh, it's stuffy in here. Maybe we need to clean your air conditioner.' This helped me realise that my feelings

CHAPTER 30

were only from the stuffiness of the room, and weren't a panic attack. My air conditioner was cleaned that day and the feelings left. This made me more aware of how my body reacted to my environment. When flying on a plane, I would feel closed in – to help me cope, I played music (yes, Phil Collins) and only used one earpiece, in my left ear. Why just my left ear? Well, that's the side that suffered from hyperacusis, and the music served as a type of distracting 'white noise'. I still feel claustrophobic on flights, but I now understand that it's caused by the air pressure. Knowing this helps me to relax a little more and not feel as panicked.

In 2010, the time finally came for the court case for work. I was to be called as a financial witness, and I was to help all of the other witnesses with their statements and be there to support them all. If you have ever been in court, you will understand the associated stress and all of the goings on. On the last day, my car decided to make a terrible noise on my way to court. I rang my mechanic, who listened to the noise and advised me to put my car on a tow truck and bring it over. I booked the tow truck and went inside the courthouse to wait. The driver messaged me on arrival, and I popped out from courthouse to unlock my car. However, as the driver was pulling my car up onto the truck, I jokingly yelled out with my arms up, 'No, don't take my car, I'll pay for the parking!' The driver's head shot around so quickly and I couldn't stop myself from laughing. Everyone in the carpark looked at us. I said, 'Sorry, I've been in court all week, I couldn't help myself. It's made me a little crazy.' He laughed with me and said he totally understood. We chatted while I signed for my car and he then took it off to my mechanic. The moral of the story is this: 'Don't mess with someone who has been in a courtroom for a week.'

Chapter 31

The year 2011 didn't start very well. Cyclone Yasi, which was a category 5 cyclone, hit our coastline, with the eye passing slightly north of us in Townsville. We were OK, but so many families lost their homes. When the roads were cleared, we packed our car with milk, bread, sanitary items, cold drinks and sweets for the rescue workers and headed north to check on our friends in Tully. We have a wonderful community here and we all pitched in to help.

Our year didn't get much better. Our son Kyle, in Perth, rang me on Mother's Day (which was 8 May that year) and had sent me a lovely bunch of flowers and a bottle of wine. We had a wonderful long chat and he told me that he loved me. The next morning, 9 May 2011, we got the phone call that every parent dreads. 'Your son has been involved in an accident at work.' My heart sank, or maybe stopped beating for a second or two. Roland and I both froze while we waited for more information. Our oldest two sons were working together as riggers for mines in Western Australia. All we knew was that half a tonne of chain had fallen off of a telehandler forklift and hit him on the side of his head. The first-aid officer had seen to him straight away and she had rung the Flying Doctor service. They now had Kyle and were taking him to Port Hedland, where the doctors would relieve the pressure in his head. The Flying Doctor service would then take him straight to Sir Charles Gairdner Hospital in Perth for surgery.

Our world was falling apart. I emailed my boss the details and asked to take immediate holidays. Roland rang Qantas and begged for us to be put on the next flight to Perth, telling staff that we needed to see our son before his surgery, in case he didn't make it. When the Qantas staff heard the reason for our request, they went above and beyond to make sure Roland, Jaiden and I got on that flight. We had under two hours to get to the airport. In that time, we sorted out care for our animals, picked up Jaiden from school and were all packed (taking our diary, phone, computer, and a few days' worth of clothes), and our friends turned up to drive us to the airport. I also grabbed Kyle's favourite soft toy from when he was little. I had kept it in my display cabinet but at that time, more than ever, I needed to hold it. Off we went to the airport, with Roland ringing them because we were running late. They told us not to worry; someone would be there to check in our bags and the plane wouldn't leave without us. We arrived and ran into the airport, and were quickly escorted onto the plane where everyone was quietly waiting for us. I'm sure, from the looks on our faces, that they all understood the reason for the delay.

Staff on the flight were supportive and made sure that we had drinks and food, as well as a supportive hand on our shoulder, which we so needed. I drew all my strength to stay calm and to try to reach my son's mind. I kept saying to him that we were on our way and to be strong. I don't know if it was my mind or if it was real, but I heard Kyle's voice say, 'Mum, I am strong and I will be OK.' For the seven-hour flight, I kept giving him my strength, thinking positively and willing him to survive. I cry while writing this because the emotion is still so raw and painful.

Roland had phoned a Brisbane-based friend who rang a church in Western Australia to organise for a local pastor to meet us at the airport. He would help to get us to the hospital. Kyle's boss also met us at the airport and we all rushed to the hospital. The staff at the hospital were expecting us, and the Flying Doctors had already landed with Kyle. His beautiful fiancée Lauren was already there with her parents and our oldest son. We held each other and waited while the staff finished the handover from the Flying Doctor service to the hospital. As soon as that was done, we were allowed to see Kyle. We walked into the room, and there was my 6ft 4in son lying on a bed with a large bandage on his head. He was connected to machines and there was a machine breathing for him. All I wanted to do was pick him up and hold him, just as I had done when he was

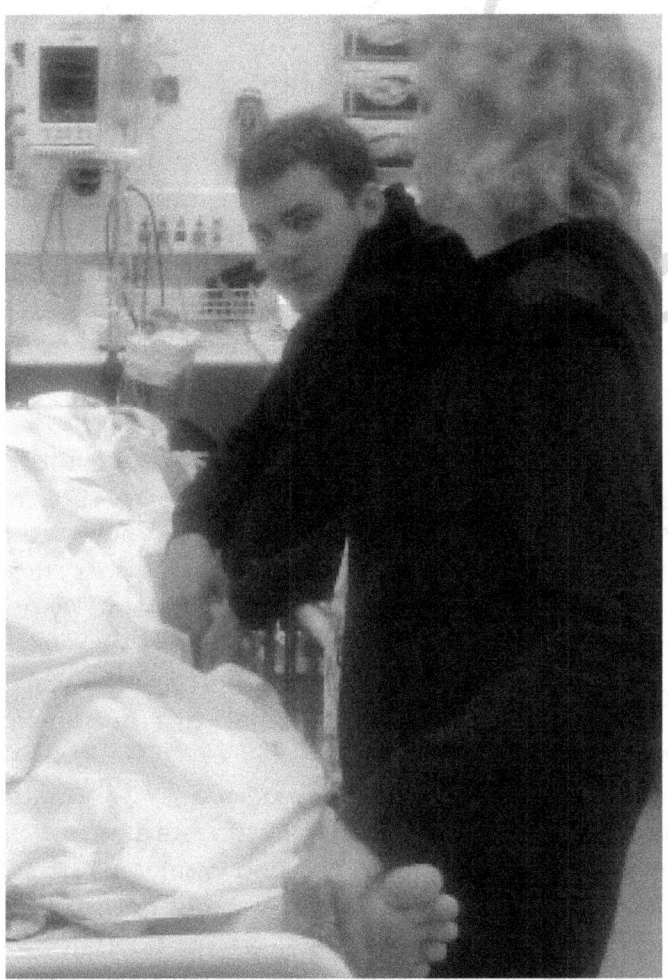

Distraught Tyrnan and I, praying for Kyle before they took him to theatre

little. Staff were preparing everything for Kyle's surgery while giving us the time we needed with him. We held his hand and gently touched his arm.

We watched them wheel Kyle away to surgery and we were shown to the waiting room. There is one thing that I want to say about Sir Charles Gairdner Hospital – they had wonderful caring staff. At one of the worst times of our lives, the staff continually popped in to give us updates, and later they were so wonderful and supportive. We knew that our son was in safe hands. When the surgeon came in to talk to us about Kyle's injury and the intended surgery, we all got to ask questions. He told us that Kyle may die in surgery. The room went quiet. I had to speak, and asked, 'What if you don't do the surgery?' The surgeon gave me such a caring look and said, 'He will die without the surgery.' I stood up, walked over to that young doctor, stood in front of him, touched his arm and said, 'Please do your best and look after my son.' He looked into my eyes and said, 'I will.' I replied with a heartfelt thank you, with tears running down my cheeks.

The staff kept us up to date with Kyle's progress throughout the surgery, and when we saw them getting his post-surgery room ready, we knew that he was still alive at that point. By now one of Tyrnan's best mates, Brett, had flown to Perth to be with us. Brett told us that Kyle was like a brother to him and he wanted to be there to support us, too. We needed that extra person who wasn't family, but who felt like family, with us.

Surgery was a success, and they placed Kyle into a coma. We were able to go in to see him. The ICU staff were angels – they looked after Kyle and made sure we understood what was happening and why. We were told we could ask as many questions as we wanted to, even if we'd asked them before. We all felt included and we trusted these people. One day Kyle's surgeon walked past and as I looked up at him he said, 'You got your wish.' I replied with a heart-filled thank you.

You can imagine how many times we walked through the hospital to get to our son's room. So many signs and pictures adorned the walls. They helped us find our way around the hospital, through all of its corridors, floors and wards. One day, a certain frame caught my eye. I'd seen it many times but never read it. On this particular day it seemed to stand out, so I stopped to read it:

CHAPTER 31

'We are not the same persons this year as last; nor are those we love. It is a happy chance if we, changing, continue to love a changed person.'

These words, by W Somerset Maugham, were words I needed at that moment. How true they were for both my son and me. I took a photo of the words to help me remember them.

Every day, Kyle seemed to be getting better and better. They started bringing him slowly out of the coma. I felt so loved when he woke briefly on my birthday, which was 10 days after the accident, to wish me a happy birthday. He also looked up at me and whispered, 'Thank you.' I knew it meant thank you for being there, talking to me, believing in me and loving me. My beautiful boy was going to be OK; it was true.

The company Kyle worked for had rented a unit for us near the hospital and given us a car so that we could get to the hospital daily. I had also spoken to the flying doctor – Annemarie van der Walt – who had looked after him on that flight. Annemarie is a very special flying doctor to our family and we have kept in contact with her over the years.

One day we were allowed to take Kyle in his wheelchair to the gardens, which were on one of the levels of the hospital building. It was here where Kyle surprised us all, because until that point he had been having so much trouble with his memory. He said, 'I'm getting married in January.' Oh, he remembered! We all looked over at Lauren. She had gone through so much and we all wanted their marriage to happen. It was a goal for Kyle to work towards. We all helped to make it happen.

After two weeks, Roland and Jaiden had to return home, but I wasn't going anywhere until my son was out of hospital. I had our oldest son to look after me and I spent every day at the hospital. I saw Kyle take his first steps when learning to walk as a child, and then his first steps when learning to walk again after his injury. I listened to his words and tried to help him remember what he was trying to say. I hugged him and wished I could make everything better. A month went by and Kyle was then in recovery, almost ready to go home. It was time for me to go back home to Townsville. There was a lot we needed to do (including preparing for Kyle's and Lauren's wedding and catching up on work) but we'd be back just after Christmas to celebrate the wedding – and what a beautiful wedding it was.

I'LL DO IT MYSELF

They say it helps to write things down, so as I flew home alone, I wrote this poem:

A Poem to My Son

Today I held my son's hand
Not knowing if it would be for the last time
I kissed him softly
Telling him I loved him
And that I'd be here when he wakes

His life was now in the hands of the doctors
And his love is in my heart

You see, he'd received a head injury at work
We flew 7000km to be by his side

The doctors did their best
But we didn't know if he'd wake up

Hours and days we waited, sitting beside him
Holding his hand and telling him we loved him and all would be fine

Days later he started to move and slowly wake
Soon I was able to look my son in the eyes and tell him
As I had many times before
'I love you'

His determination amazes everyone
Today he stands tall
As I hold him in my arms, all 6ft 4in, I tell him I love him
He tells me, 'I love you too, Mum. Thank you'

It's a thank you for everything
All those moments beside him as he slept
All those things I reassure him of
All the praise and belief
All the love and just for being his mum

Today I hold my son's hand

by Sandra Hubert, for my son Kyle
xxx

Chapter 32

My grief didn't stop with Kyle's accident. Two months later I got a phone call from my sister Joanne to let me know that our beautiful grandma had passed away after a fall. I don't know if you can relate to this, but every time I think of my grandma, I smile. I may have tears running down my face, but I am smiling. Every memory is beautiful and she left such an impression on my life that I can only smile through my tears. My sister and I planned her funeral, and what Grandma would wear. We also chose what our mother, who was living in a home with dementia, would wear. While selecting a dress for Mum, Joanne and I heard the song 'A Groovy Kind of Love' (by Phil Collins) on the department store speaker. I said, 'Joanne, listen to this song!' Her reply was, 'It's Grandma telling us this is the right dress for Mum.' It was a lovely moment.

I wrote Grandma's eulogy and we picked out special photos together to show everyone. Joanne and I knew her so well that all of the decisions for her funeral were easy for us to make. The day before the funeral, we visited the chapel for a private viewing. We placed cards and photos in the coffin with Grandma and pinned a corsage on her blouse. At that moment, 'A Groovy Kind of Love' was playing in the chapel. It was so beautiful and not planned at all. (We now consider it to be Grandma's song, and it often happens to be playing when I need an emotional lift. I think of cuddling my grandma, and of her smile and her love.)

Our mum didn't really understand what was happening on the day of the funeral, but Joanne and I held her hand and kept her close. We thanked our awesome husbands for doing the service readings for us, and we thanked our family and friends for supporting us on that day.

The love and the words of my grandma are with me always. When I have to make a decision, I often say, 'What would Grandma do?' She always did the right thing and I was so blessed to have had her for 48 of her 92 years. I treasured every moment.

At this time, I realised that I would love to work more with people who had disability. I loved my accounting work, but what if I could do both? I contacted our local TAFE to do the Certificate IV in Disability. I was able use the RPL (required prior learning) exemption instead of going to classes, and I was tested by way of assignments. When you love something, it is so easy to write about it. I completed all 15 subjects in four months, graduating on 19 July 2012. I was working full time and attending all of my committee and board meetings, but this was my passion and I enjoyed every subject – plus, I had real-life experience in each of them.

The business I had been working for was being dissolved, which gave me more time to do both private accounting and disability work. I completed day courses with titles such as Positive Behaviour Support, Active Support, Governance, and Risk Management. (Later, in 2015, I completed my Certificate IV in Work Health & Safety and I also looked into doing a rehabilitation and return to work coordinator course). I wanted to give back and make a difference in other people's lives. I understood more than most what it was like not to be yourself and to strive to get better.

Chapter 33

I had an awesome year in 2013, not only because I celebrated my 50th birthday in style with a Golden Logies-themed celebration, but because we were blessed with our first grandchild – a beautiful little girl. Our world was looking wonderful. All of our sons had amazing wives or partners and the next stage of our life had begun. My birthday was the best time to thank all of my fantastic family and friends for being there for me. For the party, I chose the right venue and I had a presenter, photographer, gold Logies and a video clip for each nominee, featuring photos and music. It was a fun evening and I still enjoy visiting my friends at their homes and seeing their gold Logies proudly sitting on shelves.

Over the next few years I also saw our hard work at Mental Illness Fellowship North Queensland become real, with the start of construction for our multi-million-dollar mental health hub. Roland and I painted a spade gold to use for the first turning of soil on the new building. Our board had spent many long hours, months and years making it happen. To be at the opening and to have Dr John Allan there as a VIP was just perfect. Dr Allan had seen me at my worst 19 years previously, and now, like this new building, he could see me as complete, too. With the building we would be able to help so many people who had mental health needs.

I was still working in both of my passions – accounting and disability. I had my accounting clients and my disability clients. I was the chairperson of Wee Care, president of The Cathedral School Past

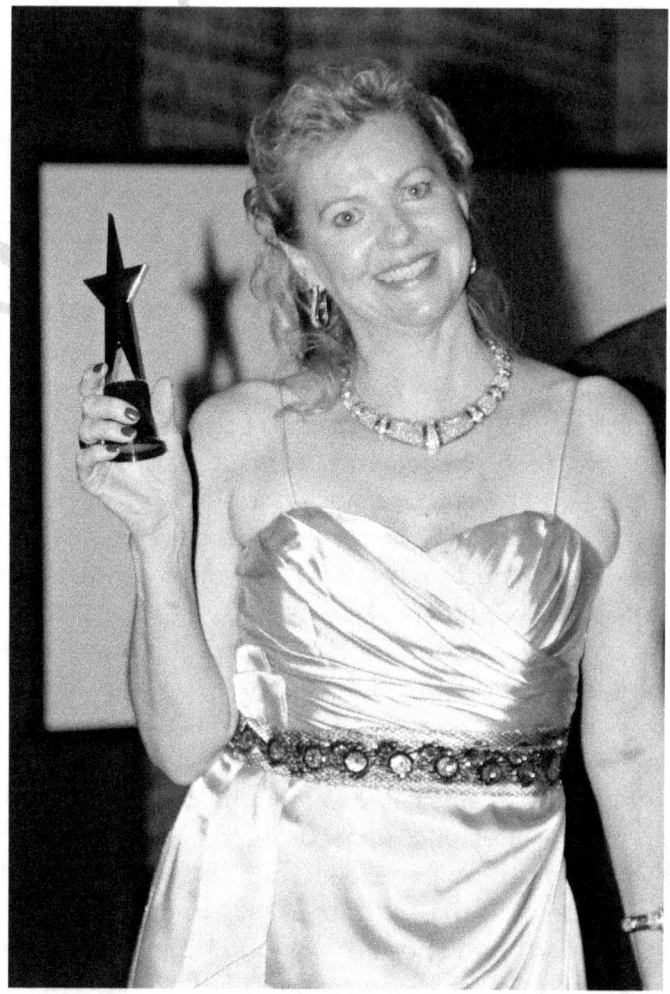
Dazzling fans and handing out awards at my 50th birthday celebration

CHAPTER 33

Students' Association, treasurer of the Monique Robinson Trust Fund and coordinator for the 'A.B.I. be in it' brain injury social group. I was also on the board of Mental Illness Fellowship North Queensland, and at our home I looked after a young girl with disabilities for a few hours a week so that her mum could have a break. I was doing all of the things that I enjoyed.

Funding opportunities were changing, so Mental Illness Fellowship North Queensland and another mental health organisation called Solas Inc started to discuss the possibility of amalgamating so that we could better serve our community. In 2018, the amalgamation resulted in a new organisation called selectability Ltd. We appointed a CEO and restructured the business model so that we could grow our footprint and help in areas of need. At our 2022 AGM we had over 3000 people relying on our services and over 600 employees, and we were in over 12 locations across North Queensland. It has been a fabulous experience to be part of this journey. In July 2018 I was able to achieve one more goal – I became a paid director of selectability Ltd. I had volunteered so many hours in my life, for so many different organisations, and it was very humbling to be recognised in this way by such a successful and caring company.

———

Chapter 34

You might think that after going through so much over so many years, I have it all figured out, that I'm 100% healed. However, I am still putting myself back together, and recognising the strength and beauty that has resulted from the process (remember my analogy about kintsugi bowls, where gold lacquer is used to repair breaks?). I still have my doubts and my problems. There isn't a reset button that I can push that will suddenly make me become 'me' again. Who is me? I seem to be searching for a conclusion, and I wonder if all I really want is a score, a percentage or a mark out of 100 that shows how close I am to being OK. Am I 80% OK? What does OK even mean? I have so many unanswered questions for which I have tried to find the answers. Every new task is a blank page, needing me to get out my notepad and plan every aspect. For example, if we're going away, I need to note down the dates of our journey, addresses of places we'll be visiting, our accommodation bookings, and what we'll need to take (even down to the type of suitcase required). I'll even write down that I have to organise a dog-sitter and cancel the newspaper. My recall may be slow, but I have learned that I need to give myself time. My expectations may be too high, but that is just me.

To help me in everyday life, I have become very aware of my surroundings. It also helps my memory if I create certain behaviours and structures. For instance, you could turn off the light at night and I could easily navigate around my house. I could almost prepare breakfast with my eyes blindfolded. Everything has its place, which means that I don't have to remember where a particular item is – I can just automatically put out my hand and pick it up, or walk to it. I have a legally blind girlfriend called Chris and we have fun together because I understand how to help her. My issue may be memory and hers may be eyesight, but the living skills I use are the same ones that Chris uses.

At work, I am able to write with both hands and do two things at once while coping with distractions such as phone calls and doors being opened. However, at home I don't deal as well with distractions, and have to do one thing at a time. I hate looking for things, so I have created an easy system whereby when I have to put something new away, I say to myself, 'Where would I look for this?' I try to keep things logical, because I'm a logical person. (Don't worry, I'm not perfect with this – I sometimes put things in a 'really safe place' and then promptly forget where that is. Luckily, this doesn't happen often!)

My job roles are so different and are perfect for the person I have become. As an accountant, board member and director, I am confident in the boardroom making decisions worth millions of dollars. However, I am just as confident as a disability support person, dancing down the aisle at the supermarket with my client to help them cope. Nobody sees me as a person with a disability; they see me as a professional and someone who cares and includes others. However, I see myself as a person with a disability, and I need to change that belief about myself.

I have asked many different professionals – from occupational therapists to psychologists to neurologists – where I sit on my road to recovery. They all say that I'm doing so well. But how do I measure this? When you have a cold, you know when you are feeling better. When you break your leg, you know when you are feeling better. When you have a brain injury and seem to be functioning well, there is no guideline. At the beginning of my recovery, I wanted to be 100% well. Yet, recently, in my undergraduate study in mental health at Monash University, I was very happy with a result of 93% (a high distinction) in one of my subjects. Perhaps I shouldn't be so hard on myself. I should just accept that I am doing well and leave it at that, without needing to be perfect. I have to remember where I started and how far I have come since then.

Chapter 35

In 2024, Roland and I celebrated 40 years of marriage. We have three awesome sons, three fabulous daughters-in-law and six wonderful grandchildren. We live on an acre of land, with lots of room for our grandchildren to play. It won't surprise you to learn that I am also the treasurer and secretary of our local Rural Fire Service (Roland is also a member of the brigade). Over the years, I have had many low moments when I couldn't see past the pain and the hurt, but my long-term goal – and Roland's – was to sit in our rocking chairs together as an old couple, watching our grandchildren.

We have an awesome timber swing on our patio and we often sit there with our grandchildren and enjoy being together. This wouldn't have happened if I had given up, and I *so* cherish those times … those little arms around my neck, those little voices saying, 'I love you, Nana.'

I smile as I look into the future and imagine putting up my hand once again to help out the community, but next time the club for which I nominate will be one that our grandchildren are in. All I want is to make a positive difference in people's lives.

I hope that this book helps you to understand where you are in life and to grab hold of your life and really live. Take each opportunity that comes along, and do your best in whatever you want to do. You really can rebuild your life after any challenge – I am living proof of that.

Ask yourself:

- Are you where you want to be? This could be in terms of where you live, or where you are in life – whether or not you have children, are married or single, have a home, have a career or job you like, or get to enjoy family time or participating in sport. It could just be whether or not you are confident and enjoying life.

- Do you need more information to help you to make a decision, to understand what is going to happen, or to move forward? Do you need to ask someone a question or do some research to help you get where you want to be?

- Is the activity that you are doing now, in this very moment, the right thing for you? For example, you may love your job, but perhaps tomorrow you would prefer to take time off to watch your son receive his award at school assembly?

- When you are elderly and look back on your life, what will you think?

I've kept these questions short so that, at any time, you can remember them and review where you are. When you come to a roadblock, stop, think and find a way around it. Life is full of challenges and all we need to do is find a way around them. Place your hands on your hips and give yourself confidence by saying, 'I'll do it myself.'

Enjoy the simple things in life. Hug your family and your friends. Make people smile. Embrace the broken pieces of your life and make something beautiful and strong from them.

Live the life you love …

Sandra.

Helpful Hints

If you have a brain injury, or you are the loved one or carer of someone with a brain injury, I want to help you. I want to give you basic steps for starting the healing journey.

To achieve any goal, all you need to do is take one step at a time. However, it helps if you know which steps to take. With my recovery, I had to discover each step myself, and this took patience, persistence, determination and tears. I had no guidelines, no information and no direction. All I had was my strong willpower and my independent nature. In this chapter, I hope to make it easier for you!

To help you start healing, it's important for you to take the time to find out more about yourself, and the things you want to improve. What are the areas in which you need help? I like to start with looking at the basics – this may sound easy, but I assure you that they are often more complex than you realise.

Let's begin with three questions. We'll explore these further in this chapter:

1. How are you now?
2. Where do you want to be?
3. What steps do you need to take to get there?

I love lists, and I recommend that you create lists as you go through the following questions. You can then take them with you when you visit doctors and specialists, because they will help you to remember the questions you want to ask.

1. How are you now?

It's time to note down all of the physical problems that you're encountering, as well as your behaviours and emotions, and issues with your senses, memory and social interactions.

To help you discover how you really are right now, and what your triggers may be, following is a list of areas for you to consider. Reflect on each area, and record what you observe. (I've included mention of my own experiences with some of these areas, and have provided strategies that worked for me.)

COORDINATION

This refers to balance and to spatial recognition. To test balance, stand up, close your eyes and touch your nose. Did you wobble and did you find your nose? Spatial recognition is more about being aware of your surroundings and gauging distance – to test this, try reaching out and picking up your glass of drink. Can you do so without bumping the glass?

HEARING

Are sounds too loud, too soft or too much for you? Sometimes we hear all of the noises around us at once, and this can be overwhelming. Hearing issues can cause anxiety and confusion. (As mentioned earlier in my story, to help me cope with too many sounds and with them being too loud, I listen to music through an earplug in the affected ear.)

VISION

How do you feel when you look around you? There can be a tendency to try to identify everything you see. This can overload your brain and overwhelm you, leading to anxiety. It could be that you are affected by fast movement occurring in front of you because your brain is trying to identify everything (however, it just can't do this). The resulting overstimulation can make you feel flustered, or as though you want to remove yourself from the situation. Sometimes we can suffer from double vision and headaches, and even aches at the back of the eye. These issues can be treated, so if you've experienced them then please speak to your doctor or eye specialist. These issues happened to me, and I was given exercises to strengthen the muscles around my eyes.

Distortions in your vision can also be a problem – for me, the floor and walls sometimes appeared to move like waves. This frightened me but my doctor reassured me that it was only my brain reconnecting itself. I also sometimes felt as though the earth itself moved. It felt like a very small earthquake, and it happened so quickly that it would only affect one of my steps when I was walking. It was reassuring to discover that it was just another reconnection occurring in my brain, and eventually it did stop happening. So, be on alert for sensations of this type. Ask questions. You may be very frightened of a particular sensation, but in reality it may be a positive sign that your brain is on the mend.

OLFACTION (SENSE OF SMELL)

Be sure to check for this because it took ages for anyone to pick up this issue with me. Can you recognise different smells, or can you even smell at all? If you can't smell anything, be aware of how your body reacts to the smell. I believe that when I smell something, the information goes to my brain and my body reacts to the smell, but I don't have a conscious awareness of what the smell actually is. When I smell something now, I wait for my body to react. It could react as if it is in survival mode (ie, my shoulders go up and I recoil, with a fight or flight response) if I smell something dangerous like smoke or chemicals. Or, when I smell a flower or nice perfume, my body relaxes and I smile. I have tested my theory when I cook. I smell the food I am cooking on the stove, and then I stop and give my brain and body time to react. I usually have a response along the lines of, 'This dish needs more thyme or a different spice,' and then I ask Roland to smell the food and see what he would recommend. Yes, he always agrees with my thoughts about what the dish needs. There is so much about the brain that we have yet to discover and understand.

SENSORY ISSUES

Brains have to cope with so much at a time, and you can be hyper-aware of multiple sensations that occur at the same time. Imagine watching television while sitting on a chair in the lounge. Your bare feet touch the floor and feel the coolness of the tiles or the texture and warmth of the carpet. The back of your body feels the warmth and degree of firmness of your chair. The fan is going and you hear its noise while feeling the breeze on your body. Your hair is moved by the breeze, which gives you another feeling to cope with. The television is on and you have to concentrate on the sounds, the words being spoken, the movement on the screen and the storyline. Your body has to regulate its temperature in relation to the breeze from the fan. Sometimes we don't cope with all of these sensations and we experience sensory overload. Have you noticed this in your own life?

BODY TEMPERATURE

Many of us have difficulties regulating our body temperature, so be aware that you may need to cover or uncover your arms or legs to adjust your temperature. It is a good idea to know if your body has temperature-regulation issues, and also to know if your body's temperature is higher than that of the average person – I have a higher-than-normal temperature, and I was told that if I become unwell I should inform the treating doctor of this.

FLEXIBILITY

This refers to both physical and mental flexibility. Do you have any flexibility issues when you move your body? Can you easily adjust to changes? Do you cope with interruptions and can you recall what you were doing beforehand?

SLEEP

Do you find it easy to go to sleep? Do you sleep through the night or do you wake up often? After my injury, I had to retrain myself to go to sleep. I tried counting sheep but I still struggled. I sought help through reading, which taught me a relaxation technique. Dr Frank McDonald taught me a 'three-second' breathing technique. He told me to say to myself, 'I am safe.' Then, I breathe in for three seconds, hold for three seconds and breathe out for three seconds. Please do give this technique a try, if you have trouble sleeping.

DISORIENTATION

Do you easily get lost or forget which direction you came from? There are various confidence-building techniques you can use to make you feel comfortable asking for help when you're lost or confused. However, you can also develop your own ways of countering disorientation. For example, I used to hate walking into a shop and then, when leaving it, not remembering how to get back to my car. I thought everyone would laugh at me if I went the wrong way. However, do you know what? Nobody even noticed. I decided that, when walking towards the shop I wanted to visit, I would take note of a nearby shop that was on the way. Then, when I left, I would stop and look for the shop I'd previously noticed, and walk in that direction. This helped me remember which way I wanted to go.

MEMORY

Do you have issues with your short-term or long-term memory? From time to time, we all forget things and can't remember names or items on our shopping list. However, when these issues affect our everyday life in a negative way, we need to look for ways to help ourselves. I write lists and have a handy notepad for writing reminders. It could be that you need to take your medication at a certain time each day – if you set up an alarm reminder on your phone, it will help you remember to do this. There are so many ways to help deal with memory issues. Write down the issues that affect you the most, and create solutions.

COMMUNICATION

This relates to what to say, how to say it, when to speak, and interacting with others. Do you understand what people are saying? How do you cope with the tone of their voice or the emotion behind the words? Do you look at facial expressions to help you understand? Do you need to give your brain time to process everything? I have a tip for you – if someone asks you a question, you can easily give your brain time to process things by saying, 'Give me a minute to think about that' or 'I'm not sure what you are asking me.'

EMOTIONS

Are you able to identify emotions that you are feeling? Sometimes, emotions can blend into each other and it can be confusing to work out how you feel. To help with this, take a moment to look at your situation – are you safe? Are voices raised? Are you in pain? Is someone else in pain? Notice how your body is positioning itself. It will reflect the emotion you are truly feeling. For example, if you are standing tall and breathing deeply, you may be feeling confident. If your shoulders are curled forwards with your arms protecting your body, you may be feeling unsafe. If your shoulders are back and your chest is protruding, you may be feeling defensive. When you see someone and you smile as you raise your hand to wave, you are most likely experiencing a happy, friendly feeling. The more you understand your reactions in different situations, the easier it will be to identify your emotions.

SOCIAL INTERACTION

Are you OK going out in public or does the thought of it overwhelm you and make you anxious? I've found it helpful to put in place strategies to cope. It could be that I have someone go out with me. Knowing the layout of the place I am going to is also a big help, as is knowing when I will be leaving, who will be there and what is happening when I am there. It might be that you only need someone to explain these things verbally, in the order in which they will happen, for you to cope well with your next social interaction. Do you find it easy to talk to others? If not, you can develop skills that will help. Learning positive words to use, and questions to ask, will make you feel more confident when holding conversations.

ANXIETY & DEPRESSION

Do you feel numb or empty, or as though there is nothing to look forward to? Do you feel paralysed at the thought of doing even the simplest things? Anxiety and depression are common for so many people, and it's OK to talk about them and seek help. They caused me lots of problems and stopped me from doing things, so I found ways to help myself and – importantly – I also sought help from doctors and psychologists. One technique that helped was to imagine that the experience of living my life was like floating down a creek. I visualised myself holding onto the sides of the creek (the sides were the issues in my life), which stopped me from floating away. I would then imagine letting go and enjoying the feeling of floating down the creek with the flow of the water, the flow of life. I've used this awesome technique for nearly 30 years. However, you need to find what works for you (and please do seek professional guidance).

GRIEF

Do you find yourself feeling exceptionally sad about your injury? Do you ruminate on it? You may well be experiencing a sense of grief, and this is completely normal. At first, I was so busy recovering that I didn't grieve for what I had lost. Looking back, I can see that I tried to deny having a brain injury. I also felt that because I survived, I could face anything. However, when I realised how close I came to death, and when I became frustrated at not being back to my old self, I hit bottom. I had to accept myself as I was so that I could move on. It was comforting to find out that all of those feelings were a normal part of the grieving process. I could also see that I had almost made my way through the stages of grief. Understanding these stages helps your recovery, and there is so much help out there. If you are going through grief, please ask for support.

ACCEPTANCE

Do you accept yourself and your injury? It's so important to do so, and choosing to accept yourself as you are can be a journey in itself. Acceptance is actually a part of the grieving process. I mentioned grieving earlier, but I've separated acceptance into its own point because it is so important. After my injury, I found it hard to accept myself because I wanted to achieve so much more. Over time, I learned to accept myself because I realised how far I had come from the first day of my illness. I reflected on what I had gone through and where I had succeeded (writing this book has helped me with this). I am truly humbled by my journey. I see that others accept me for being me and they don't judge me for my faults. So why should I be so hard on myself?

I want you to experience the feeling of freedom that self-acceptance gives you. How can you do this? By accepting who you are, what you can do and where you fit in the world. Write a list of the good things about you. For a start, you survived your injury! Perhaps you have a great sense of humour? What else? Tell me! Then write another list, this time outlining the things that you can do – can you smile, drive a car, stand on one leg? What is on your list?

ALL LEARNED BEHAVIOUR

Do you struggle with things that you used to do easily? Whether you're a person with a brain injury, a stroke victim, or a carer, friend or family member of an injured person, how do you think you would cope if you forgot basic tasks like showering yourself? I had to re-learn what seemed to be an endless list of things. When to eat. How much to eat. How it feels to need to go to the toilet. Social skills such as when to speak, what to say, how to act in public and where to sit at any event (including at the doctor). I even had to re-learn which side of the path to walk on – in Australia, we usually walk on the left side and people coming towards us pass by on our right.

Think of what we teach children from birth. There is so much for them to learn, and for us to re-learn (even though we aren't children). It helps to be aware of your body's feelings and reactions while you re-learn. For example, if I have morning tea at 10am I know that I will probably need to go to the toilet at 11am. Earlier in my recovery, I wouldn't pay attention to when I had a drink, and I'd end up busting later! Now, I notice that I feel different in my lower abdomen and I then think, 'Maybe that is my bladder feeling full.' So off I go to the toilet, and I discover that my reasoning was correct. I remember that feeling of pressure in my abdomen, and each time I feel it (as well as looking at the clock to determine when I last had a drink), I know that I need to go to the toilet. This is only one example. Earlier in my story I mentioned that I had to re-learn how to wash myself in the shower. You can imagine how many other things I had to re-learn. However, doing this can be so quick and can make life so easy.

There is so much more that I could add to this list of issues. We are all different, so please just use this as a guide. I highly encourage you to take the time to write your list, ask your questions and find answers so that you can be 'you' again. One of the best ways of coping with challenges is feeling that you have some control over your health and your life.

I remember sitting with my doctor, feeling frail, scared and anxious, and that my world was ending. She talked with me, calmed me down and told me that I had control in my life. I could make my own choices and I had every right to ask questions. By helping me realise this, she empowered me. It made me feel stronger and I knew that I could take control. I'll never forget her understanding, and I thank her.

One of my favourite sayings is that information cures fear. When I find myself worrying about something, I go and research it and find the answers.

2. Where do you want to be?

Now that you've written your list that documents 'where you're at' (in the areas I covered earlier), it's time to think about your goals. How do you really want your life to be? Your goals may be small, such as remembering to brush your teeth at night, or they may be big, such as graduating from university or learning to ride a horse. All of your goals are important and achievable. Write down every single one; everything you can think of. Seeing them written down will inspire you to find the answers to your current challenges, and it helps you to focus on the future. It feels so good to take control of your life. One goal of mine was to be able to walk my children to school on my own, and walk home, without getting lost.

3. What steps do you need to take to get there?

A goal can seem overwhelming, so let's make it easier. Just look at each goal and identify the steps you need to take to reach it – the steps can be as small or as big as you'd like.

One of my goals was to write my own story so that I could help others. I wrote notes and ideas, cried, wrote more and became consumed by the enormity of it all. It wasn't until I spoke with my publishing consultant and editor, Joanne, that I started writing the book itself. Joanne gave me the steps I needed to achieve my goal. I took it one step at a time, one page at a time.

Please take my advice – you don't have to do it alone. Find the right people to help you with each step of your recovery, and you *will* reach your goals.

I am here to help you. I may not have all the answers but I can listen and together we can find the answers. I wish you all the best.

———

PS If you would like a direct source of support and information regarding encephalitis, I highly recommend that you visit the website of non-profit Encephalitis International: encephalitis.info.

Acknowledgements

I have been blessed to have had some beautiful people in my life. My great-grandma gave me her strength and love, and also taught me not to fear death. When I was a young girl, she became bedridden after having had a stroke. I stood beside her hospital bed while she told me that she had spent the day walking through the gardens with her husband (who had passed away many years earlier). All I could see was love. If she believed that she was walking in the garden with her husband, then I knew that there was more to life than what we have here on Earth.

My awesome paternal great aunty May taught me to stand up for myself and show the world who I am. I loved her visits and I remember her telling me in the 1970s to show off my legs because nobody would want to see her old legs. She also taught me to ask questions. She had to have a medical procedure on her leg and the doctor asked if she wanted to be sedated. Great Aunty May said, 'No, I want to make sure you do the right thing.'

I grew up with the best grandparents on both sides of my family. My dad's parents – Nan and Pop – showed me what's meant by family, and the importance of being together and including others. I was one of 18 grandchildren, yet I felt special, and loved by Nan and Pop. We had so many holidays together. Pop taught me how to shoot and fish, and encouraged a love of boats and exploring.

Now I have my own home with Roland, and we carry on Nana and Pop's legacy by including everyone. Family dinners are fun nights that include our friends and our children's friends. We have all enjoyed many holidays and special times together, just like when I was a young girl. We have three children but I'm called 'Mum' by so many others. I thank you all for being part of our extended family. You all have a special place in my heart.

My mum's parents – Grandma and Poppa – were my strength. They showed me love unconditionally and made sure that I felt it. I was never judged by them; only loved. When Roland came into my life, Poppa saw how happy I was and asked Roland only one thing: 'Are your intentions honourable?' Roland replied with, 'Yes.' That was all Poppa needed to know, and he gave us our blessing. I was also shown to accept death, with Grandma telling me of her dreams and what she knew of God. She was one of eight children, and she had a dream that she walked the staircase to heaven beside each of her sisters. Every time they reached the top, God would welcome them and then say to Grandma, 'Joan, it's not your turn. Go back down the stairs.' I knew as a young girl that my grandma would be the last of her family to die. She also taught me to believe in my dreams and stand proud.

Parents are so important, and mine taught me to be like a piano – 'straight, upright and grand'. I learned to be independent, believe in myself and stand tall. My parents treated my friends like family and I have so many precious memories of fun evenings together at our home.

People come into your life for a long time or for a short time. My life has been blessed by meeting and getting to know many beautiful people. I have been enriched by their presence. They have helped me in my career and my studies, and made me stronger and able to cope better. They have shown me acceptance, challenged me, encouraged me and stood with me. It is so difficult to name everyone from the different areas of my life – friends, neighbours, work colleagues, business associates and others – but you know who you are. Many of you went above and beyond to help over the years and I thank you so much.

A huge thank you to the health professionals who crossed my path – among them, all of the ambulance officers, specialists, nurses, admin staff, doctors, neurologists and psychologists, and my anaesthetist and psychiatrist. Thank you for your part in saving my life and helping in my recovery. I appreciate all of you.

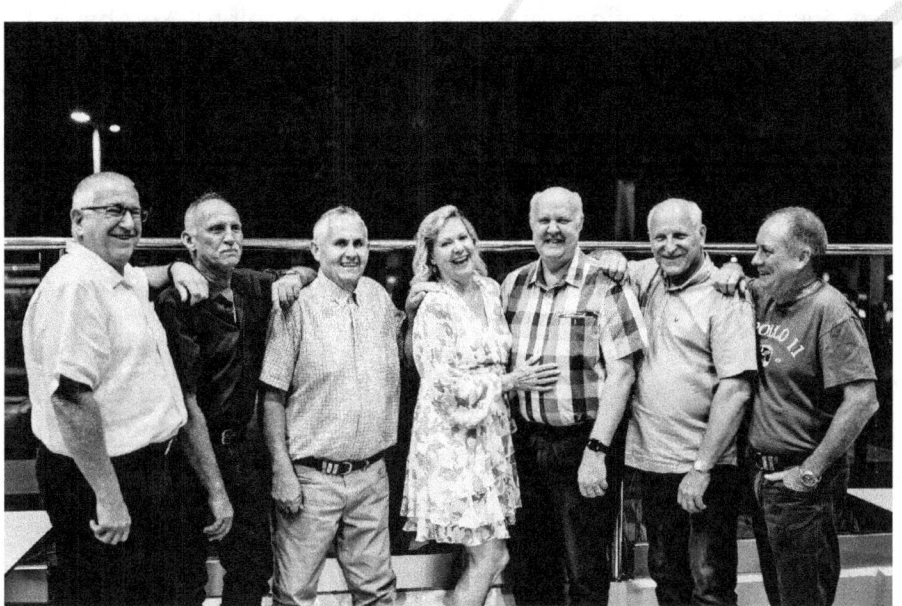
Peter, Roland, Wayne, me, Barry, Craig and Scott – friends for a lifetime

A special mention to my dear friends of over 40 years. Peter, Wayne, Barry, Craig and Scott, we have all been there for each other over the years. I have so many wonderful memories of times both happy and sad that we have faced together. Thank you for being part of my life, and of Roland's life. Our friendships are each one of a kind and I will treasure them always. I love you all, and may our friendships last forever.

To my awesome editor, Joanne Newell. Thank you for sharing this journey of writing my book with me. You have been so supportive, encouraging, patient, understanding and helpful. You have the ability to ask me the right questions, the ones that make me really understand my true feelings and emotions and express those in my story. I was able to share with you my darkest times and happiest moments, and I knew you wouldn't judge me. It was as if you could see it all through my eyes and emotions. I thank you so much for not giving up on me and for helping me to achieve yet another goal, that of writing my own book. I did it! (With your help, may I add.) Thank you.

My husband, Roland, is my everything. He completes me and is my biggest supporter. Together, we can face anything. We talk about everything, laugh at the silliest thing, and enjoy just being together – holding hands, being in the moment, and not needing to speak. Forty years after meeting, we both still feel the same connection. Roland, I thank you for being you and loving me so much. You are my shoulder to cry on, my backbone with which to stand up, my support, my strength, my love and my life. Without you, I don't think I would cope. You have brought laughter into my life, made dreams come true and stood by me. You don't even mind being referred to as 'Sandra's husband' at functions. We love each other completely and can share anything.

Family is so important, and I thank them all for the love and support they gave me throughout my recovery. To my three sons who have held me and told me that they love me – I have watched you all grow to become men, to marry and to have your own families. I'm proud of you and I love you with everything that I am. I'm here for you and your wives and I'll worry about you till the day I die. I cherish all of my grandchildren and I love seeing them grow, feeling their hugs and hearing them say, 'I love you, Nana' – another dream come true.

ACKNOWLEDGEMENTS

To our grandchildren, Olivia, Eva, Anastasia, Wynter, Harvey and Stella. I wish you all the best in life and I will love you forever.

I am eternally thankful to be alive.

Live, laugh and love ...

———————————

About Sandra

Sandra Hubert is a 'people person' with a big heart. Ask anyone who knows her. They'll tell you that she lives life to the fullest, pouring love on family and friends and celebrating life at every chance.

A serious brain injury in 1994 threatened to take away the life she loved, but she simply refused to give up. There was too much to live for. She put her hands on her hips, tipped her nose in the air, and said, 'I'll do it myself.'

She's come so far since then – she works as a carer and on boards of community organisations; makes memory cards and sews memory pillows and teddies for grieving families; and brings accountancy skills to businesses in her home city of Townsville, Queensland.

When not giving to her community, Sandra loves nothing more than spending time with husband Roland and their amazing sons, daughters-in-law and grandchildren; enjoying beautiful roses from her garden; clinking glasses of Champagne with friends old and new on camping trips; stepping out in a pair of glam high heels from her colourful collection; and swaying to the music of Phil Collins.

This 'people person' is so grateful to have been given a second chance – life really is too short.

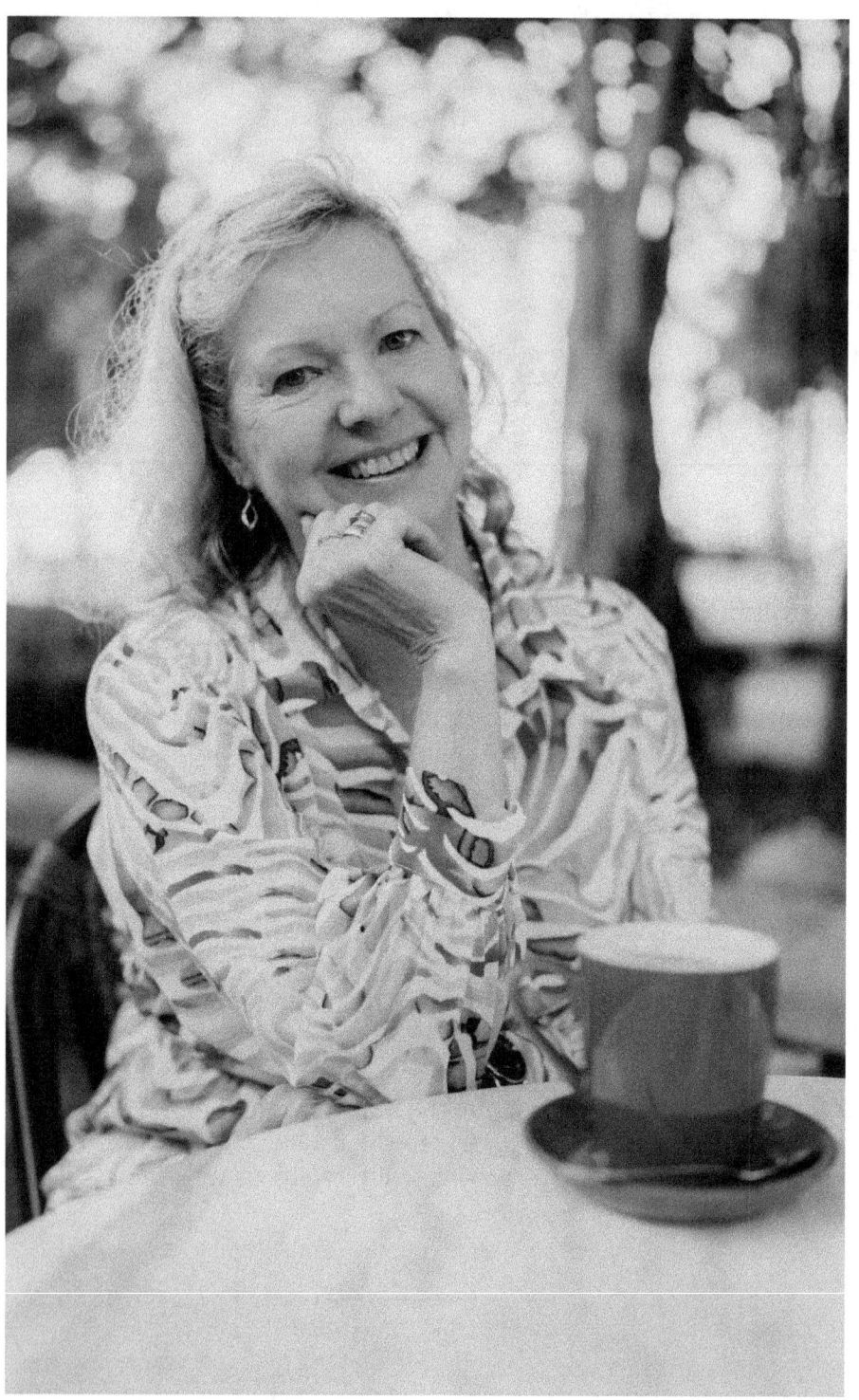

MENTORING MAGIC

Sandra Hubert is not a therapist.

However, she's been through *a lot* in her life,
and she has deep empathy.
'Helping people' is her love language.

If you're struggling with something – illness, recovery, heartbreak, loss, loneliness or plain old unhappiness – please know that Sandra is here for you.

Book a mentoring call with her and experience
what it's like to really be heard.

You'll be free to share your troubles,
and together you'll start looking
at the bright side of life and creating strategies
to help you through your situation.

Head over to Sandra's website
to get the ball rolling:

sandrahubert.com

———

Review Request

Dear Reader

I would appreciate it if you could share your thoughts with others by leaving a review.

To leave a review simply go to the review section on the amazon.com page for *I'll Do It Myself*. Click on the big button that says, 'Write a customer review' and enter your star rating and written review.

Thank you so much ...

Sandra.